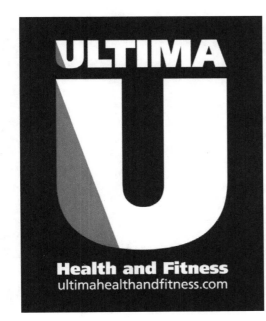

ULTIMA HEALTH AND FITNESS

ULTIMA HEALTH AND FITNESS

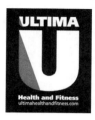

Written by
Douglas Graham Fulford - Certified General Accountant. C.G.A.

Edited by Stephanie Elisabeth Fulford – Master of Arts - Communications

Photography by Bernard Clark www.bernardclark.com

Book Layout & Interior Design by Kaitlyn Kribs | CMYKait Graphics

Graphics Book Cover by Halton Signs

Published by Douglas Fulford, June 2011

Disclaimer Notice

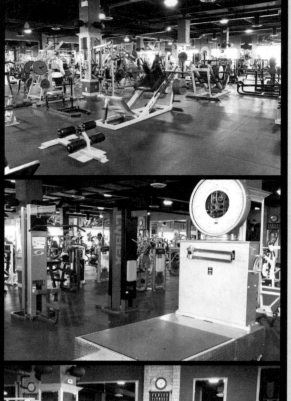

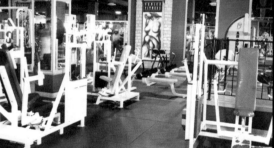

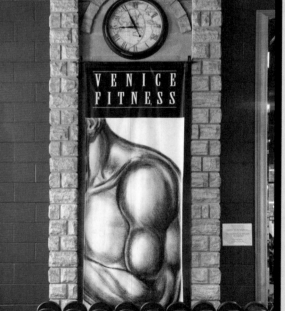

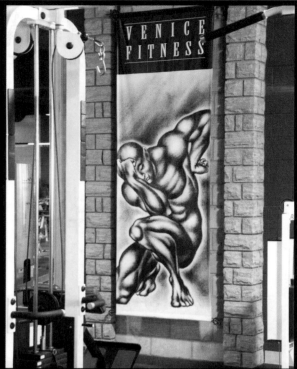

Fitness
Photography
by
Bernard Clark
www.bernardclark.com

taken at:

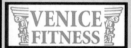

750 Warden
Ave.
Toronto
M1L 4A1
416-752-8364

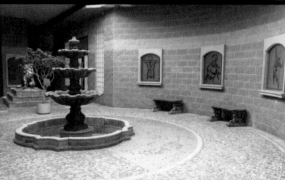

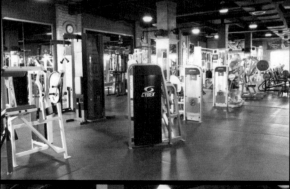

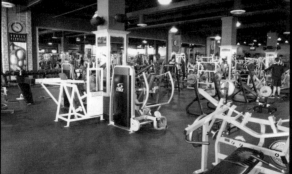

ULTIMA POEM DEDICATION

"That's the Way Life Is"

Adapted from a Rhythm & Blues Song from the 1960's

As the bitter tears fall from your eyes
A thousand times you ask yourself why
The ones you loved have departed
And you're left alone, and broken hearted
Life just comes and goes
How long it lasts nobody knows
But now's the time to be strong
And just remember, now that they're gone
That's the way life is

I know you're walking down a lonely road
And your heart carries a heavy load
I know you feel that you haven't got a friend
And your whole world is caving in
You wish that you had never been born
Now that you're alone to weep and mourn
But now's the time to be strong
And just remember, now that they're gone
That's the way life is

Life can be a hurting thing
Or it can be warm as a breath of spring
When loved ones are present, everything is all right
But when they're gone, you can't sleep at night
The road of life is rough sometimes
Don't let it get the best of you
I've been hurt by life too
I know just what you're going through
But now's the time to be strong
And just remember, now that they are gone
That's the way life is

Life is here today, and gone tomorrow
All filled with joy, then turns to sorrow
One day gladness, the next day sadness
That's the way life is
That's the way life is

ULTIMA HEALTH AND FITNESS

CHAPTER SUMMARY

Introduction : "Mr. Fulford, you have a broken back"

Dedications and Acknowledgements

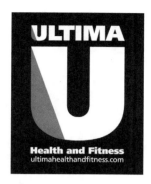

INTRODUCTION

"MR. FULFORD, YOU HAVE A BROKEN BACK."

When I regained consciousness, I found myself strapped to a stretcher with two paramedics carrying me to the ambulance. I was in great pain for several hours. After undergoing numerous x-rays and a cat scan, the doctor reported that I had fractured three vertebrae in my lower back, and suffered a concussion. I held out hope that my injury was not as serious as the doctor reported; I could not believe what had taken place that day. I had fallen about 10 feet from a main floor into the basement and landed squarely on my back. The previous three years of my life had been very chaotic: three career changes, eleven house moves (which included my daughter and mother in law), and two deaths in the family. My stress level was right off the charts and this accident seemed to cap off a run of misfortune. What else could go wrong? I felt both helpless and hopeless as I lay in bed for hours at home over several weeks. Having a shower and getting dressed was an "event" during those dark days.

But there was no surgery and the bones healed perfectly after three months, leaving me with soft tissue damages to overcome. My previous 18 years of dedication to health and fitness paid huge dividends in my rapid recovery. Within six months, I was back to the gym and training almost as hard as I had before the accident. Despite the fact that I was 65 years old, the recovery was that of someone in their 20s – or so I was told by the specialists I frequented.

The accident left me immobile for a few weeks and it was during this time of reflection that I decided to produce this book as a tribute to the benefits of good health and fitness. I hope that you will be motivated by this book to permanently change your lifestyle and ultimately improve your own health and fitness level.

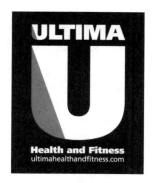

CHAPTER

1

A HISTORY OF THE AUTHOR AND HOW MAJOR TRAUMAS CHANGED HIS DIRECTIONS IN LIFE

THE EARLY DAYS

Thinking back on my childhood, I have nothing but fond memories of endless days spent playing with my brother both inside and outside our home. Most often, one of my parents would have to search out the neighborhood to locate us and make us come home to bed. My brother and I were inseparable and we had a very close-knit family who enjoyed our time together. My brother and I used to do crazy stunts like grab onto moving car bumpers in the winter to slide on the snow in our leather sole shoes. It was great until we hit a dry patch of road, and then of course we went flying. It was a wonder we were not seriously injured in such pranks, but back then we did not realize the foolishness of such actions. I did dodge my first bullet at about age 12 when I was swimming and lost consciousness due to exhaustion. I slipped under the water and remained there for several minutes. When someone finally noticed that I was missing, they began to look for me. When they finally found me, they dragged me to the shore but could not get a heartbeat. They performed CPR and called the police who took me to the hospital where I subsequently recovered. I had another close call when I raced my bike at full speed toward one of the busiest streets in Toronto and then hit my brakes in an attempt to skid the bike sideways onto the sidewalk just before I came to the street. Unfortunately, the chain came off the sprocket and I rocketed straight out onto the street into busy traffic. Once again, I dodged another bullet and I was very lucky not to be hit by a car. There are many more stories of crazy adventures with my brother and friends that are etched in my memory and all of them bring a smile to my face. I had a great childhood, which helped me to prepare for the many challenges that lay ahead in my life.

My mother was a kind, loving, caring, and gentle woman who provided the foundation for a warm, stable and supportive family. She went about life with a quiet and patient (though determined) resolve to achieve her goals in life. Family and friends meant everything to her. She always made a special effort to maintain contact and harmony with everyone she knew. My dad was a hard working man who, though not highly educated, managed to improve his job positions as time went by. He had a mischievous nature, which I inherited, and he loved to laugh and play his piano at social gatherings in our home where all would join in and sing to his music. Life was as good as it gets.

That all changed on June 7, 1959, when my mom was killed by a drunk driver who went through a stop sign late at night, with no lights, and broadsided my parents car. For those of you who might consider drinking and driving an individual choice without consequence, you need to know that the pain and sorrow of losing a family member or loved one due to the negligence of a drunk driver never goes away. Please don't drink and drive under any circumstance. My dad was badly hurt, but survived, and came to see my brother, my sister and I the very next day despite his injuries, to provide solace. My brother and I were totally devastated and we were like lost sheep without

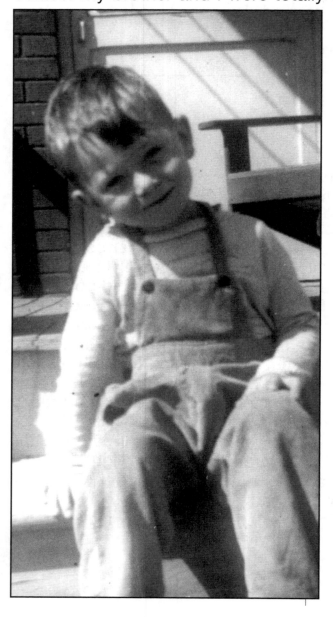

our mom for love and guidance. My poor father had buried his own father just six months to the day that same year, and only 7 years before he found his mother who had taken her life in a gas stove in our family home. Now he had two young boys and a five month old daughter to care for on his own. I look back now and realize the tremendous stress all of those events must have caused him. We went through a series of live-in care givers that never really worked well and eventually my father married one of the care givers. The marriage was a disaster, and there was constant unease and tension in our home. I had great difficulty concentrating in school and as a result I never graduated from high school. At age 17, I packed all my worldly belongings on my 3-speed bike and ran away from home, riding over 500 kilometers to Montreal in three days. I was caught by police in Montreal and was held in jail for a few days on a vagrancy charge for a few days before my father came to take me by train back to Toronto. Did I mention the bike had one of those narrow racing saddles? Needless to say, by the time I got to Montreal, I was a soprano! I never returned home, but ended up supporting myself by working in a pizzeria for over 30 hours a week for only $0.75 per hour, while also attending school. I finally got my second last year of high school completed after three attempts, and decided to get into the work field.

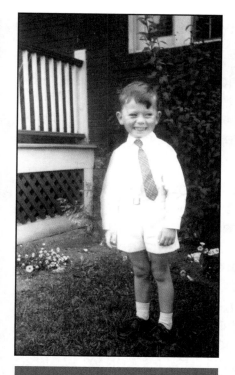

ONE HAPPY KID

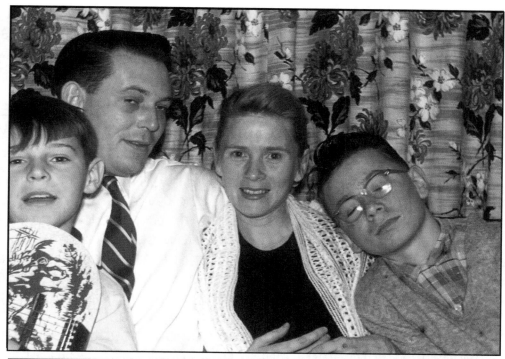

A HAPPY, HARMONIOUS, PEACEFUL FAMILY FILLED WITH LOVE - A CHILD COULD NOT ASK FOR MORE

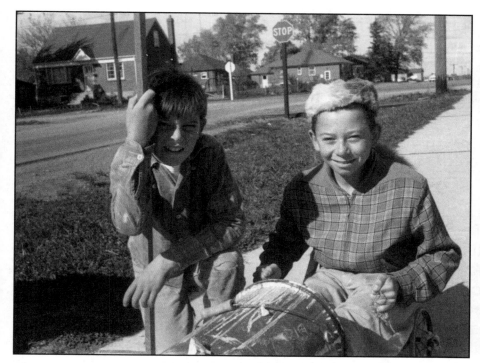

RACING HOMEMADE "CRATES" WITH BROTHER BOB

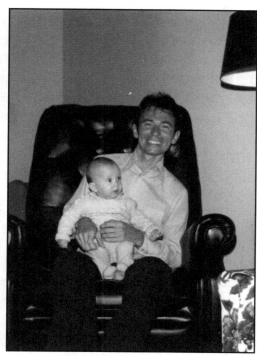

DOUG AS A YOUNG MAN

ENTERING ADULTHOOD

The next few years were devoted to working as a clerk and spending all my money on cars and clothes. I was speed crazy, and I had a series of high performance cars. They included: a Bug Eyed Austin Healy Sprite with a small block Chevy engine, a pristine 1957 Chevrolet Belair two-door hardtop with a small block Chevy engine, a 1964 Corvette convertible with a 327-365 horsepower engine, a 1970 Chevelle SS with an LS6 450 horsepower engine, and three different Jaguar XKE roadsters, amongst many more. If I had kept only a couple of those cars, I could have retired very comfortably today.

I also loved to play sports, and though I was not very talented, I enjoyed the many hours spent with friends playing football, hockey, and racing Go Karts. During my years as a young adult, playing sports was the time when I felt most relaxed and happy. Dating was really tough for me. I had very low self-esteem and I was absolutely petrified to approach women, so there was not much happening in that area of my life until my later 20s when I became more comfortable around the opposite sex. Along the way, I needed some professional counseling from a psychiatrist to help me overcome my shyness and insecurity. For those of you suffering the same ailment, there is no shame in getting some professional help to overcome your doubts. Remember that health and fitness extends into your emotional and psychological wellbeing, and just as you may need help in the gym to overcome physical barriers, help in the area of emotional difficulties can provide you with the balance necessary to have a fulfilling life overall.

Since I did not have a high school diploma or University degree, I felt I needed to pursue a higher education in order to progress in my career. I began the Certified General Accountant (CGA) course while I was working. It was very tough and I struggled every step of the way. Concentration and studying are not my strengths and there were many times when I just wanted to quit the course out of frustration and because of my inability to grasp the subjects. But I persevered and after 10 years of part-time studies, I finally got my CGA degree at the age of 38. Once again, to those of you who are struggling with academics or other obstacles in your life, hard work and perseverance - together with a little guidance from a mentor - will get you through. Please do not give up. As I discuss later in the book, perseverance is an especially important quality when it comes to your health and fitness.

It was during the initial years of working and taking my CGA that I dodged my next two bullets. I was working two full time jobs to pay for the cars that I was buying. One of the two jobs was driving a taxi at night until 1:00 AM, and I had to rise at 7:30AM to go to my day job. By the time I arrived home at 1:00 AM, I was understandably exhausted. At the time, my roommate and I shared an attic in an old house in downtown Toronto. He was a night hawk and would sleep during the day. One night, he returned around 2:00AM to change clothing and accidentally left a cigarette burning on his night table by his bed. To this day, I do not know what woke me up. I thought that I was having a nightmare and stumbled down the staircase to our common kitchen. I sat there for a while to catch my thoughts and then headed back to the attic. When I opened the door, a huge cloud of white smoke came out and I realized the place was on fire. I banged on another tenant's door to wake him up. When he saw the smoke, he panicked, but had enough sense to call 911. He then proceeded to say, "come quick – we have a big fire here," and then hung up the phone. I had to remind him that he needed to give an address. The fire truck arrived after his second call and put out the fire. Fortunately the damage was minor, but I was pretty shaken up by the incident. When my roommate arrived home, he expressed shock at what had happened but his main concern was that his best sweater had been burned up. I knew right then that it was time to get a place on my own. While I was at the same rooming house, and working the two jobs, I came home one evening from my day job and threw a TV dinner in the stove. I only had 30 minutes to eat and get to the taxi stand. I turned on the stove but the stove pilot light was out and I cursed and ran upstairs to get some matches. When I got back, I opened the stove door, lit the match, and was promptly blown across the room from the explosion. I lost my eyebrows and eyelashes, but survived to tell another story.

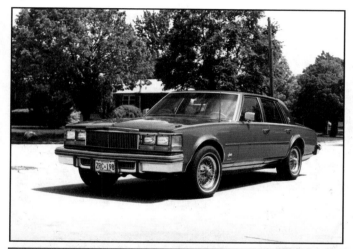

1979 CADILLAC SEVILLE ELEGANTE; IT NOW RESIDES IN BEVERLY HILLS CALIFORNIA

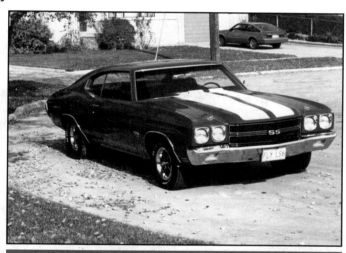

1970 CHEVELLE SS 454 LS6 450 HORSEPOWER - THIS CLASSIC MUSCLE CAR NOW RESIDES IN LAS VEGAS

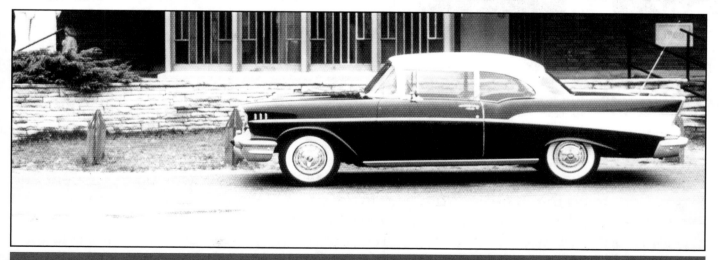

1957 CHEVROLET FROM CALIFORNIA; IT WAS ABSOLUTELY PRISTINE

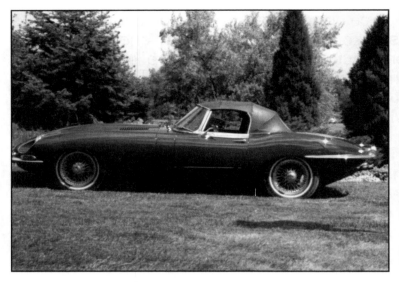

1968 JAGUAR XKE ROADSTER - A TIMELESS SPORTS CAR

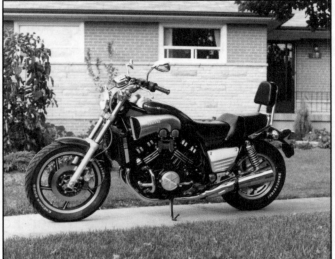

1985 YAMAHA V MAX - MY VERY FIRST MOTORCYCLE - IN IT'S DAY, THE FASTEST PRODUCTION BIKE IN THE WORLD

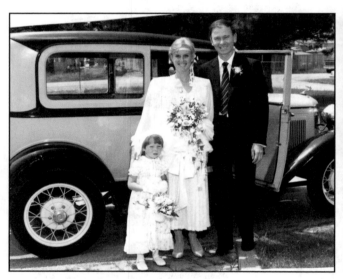

1928 MODEL A FORD TUDOR - PERFECT FOR THE WEDDING

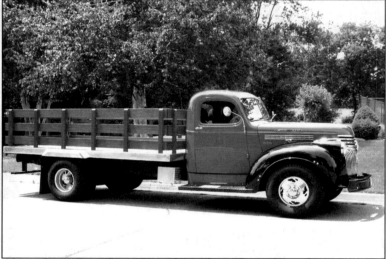

1946 CHEV 3 TON DUALLY - OFF THE ORIGINAL HOMESTEAD OF MY ANCESTOR DANIEL PRETTY BORN IN 1794

A FAMILY LIFE

I finally settled down in a marriage in my early thirties. My career was on the ascent and life was becoming much easier from a financial point of view. But the marriage was not working and despite all of our efforts, my first wife and I were simply not compatible. Just prior to our separation in the latter part of our marriage, we had a beautiful daughter whom we named Julie. She was a joy to behold. Julie had an engaging smile and boundless energy and was always happy and enthusiastic from the very start. I now recall that she never complained about anything and would always make the best of any situation.

Julie was extremely gifted as a student and in her final exams for police college, she stood first in her class of 100 graduates with an average of 97.2%. I could not be any prouder. It was a painful chapter in my life when I decided to end the marriage. Julie was only one year old, and I am fortunate that she has formed a strong relationship with my current wife Annemarie and our daughter Stephanie.

I met my current wife Annemarie on a blind date. I was immediately impressed by her natural beauty and her friendly personality. She was not as impressed by me – I was not really her type. Plus, she was also just getting out of a marriage that did not work and

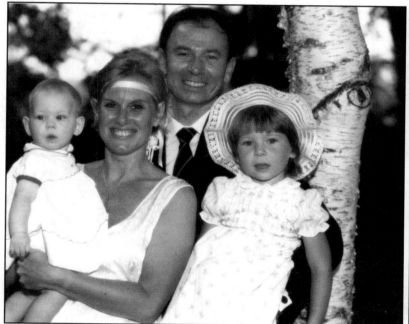

OUR WEDDING DAY WITH JULIE AND STEPHANIE

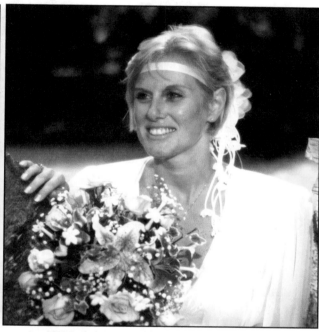

ANNEMARIE - A BEAUTIFUL BRIDE

she did not want to get seriously involved with anyone at the time. I had to show a great deal of patience and perseverance as she limited our dating and continued dating other men she considered more to her liking. She later acknowledged that it was my constant efforts to make her happy, to make her laugh a lot, and my close relationship with Julie that convinced her to give me a chance to prove myself. We became passionate lovers and Annemarie became pregnant with our daughter Stephanie. The birth of our daughter Stephanie was, in the words of Annemarie, "the greatest moment of my life". I guess that makes me chopped liver! But I do truly understand her reasons for saying those words. Stephanie turned out to be like Julie in almost every way. The two of them bonded immediately and their personalities were a mirror image. There were many occasions when friends would simply get the two girls mixed up and proceed to identify them incorrectly. I am a blessed dad, and I am so proud of both my children for their achievements and for becoming responsible adults and model citizens.

It was during these years that I took up two hobbies that used to relax me: cooking and gardening. They still play a role in my life today and there are many memories of many dinner parties that were hosted at our home for both family and friends. For me, cooking and gardening are creative outlets that have positive, healthy effects. Gardening allows

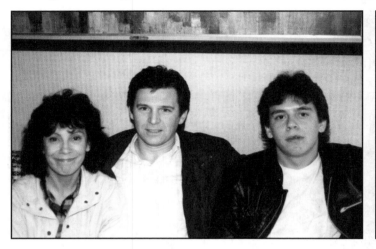

BROTHER BOB, WIFE APRIL AND SON TED - IT WAS BOB WHO PUT THE IDEA OF THIS BOOK IN MY MIND

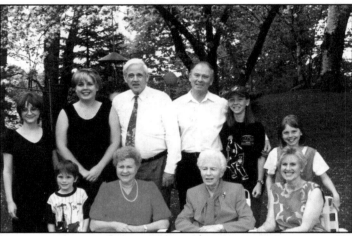

FAMILY GET TOGETHERS - A REGULAR OCCURRENCE - THE FAMILY LOVED MY COOKING

me to spend countless hours outside getting fresh air and being active, which may not appear to affect my health and fitness, but it's important to remember that even minor physical activities are superior to inactivity. Cooking has been an equally rewarding activity for me, as I am able to experiment and create meals for myself and my family,

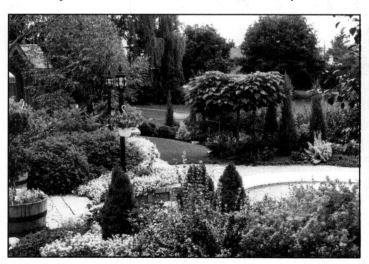

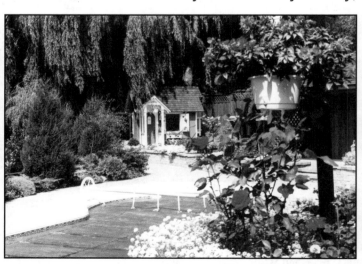

AWARD WINNING GARDENS BECAME A HOBBY THAT BROUGHT GREAT PEACE OF MIND, IN A BUSY WORK ENVIRONMENT

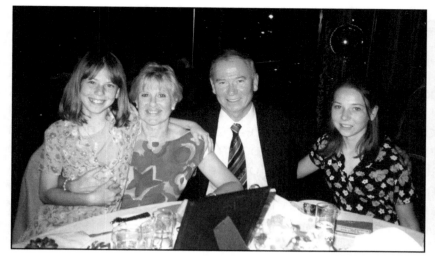

ANNEMARIE'S 50TH BIRTHDAY

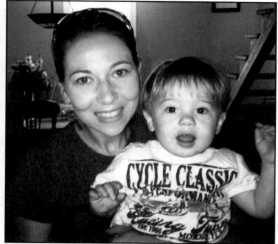

MY FIRST GRANCHILD COOPER

that I am confident are healthy and fresh and superior to the fast food that so many individuals depend on as their main food source. Healthy food is discussed later in the book in more detail.

I was now in my mid-forties and at the zenith of my business career. I had it all – a beautiful and devoted wife, two wonderful daughters, a comfortable home with an award winning landscaped back yard that I had fashioned, a good share of an established business, and a six-figure salary. I was on cloud nine, but that was all about to rapidly change. Life had another surprise in store.

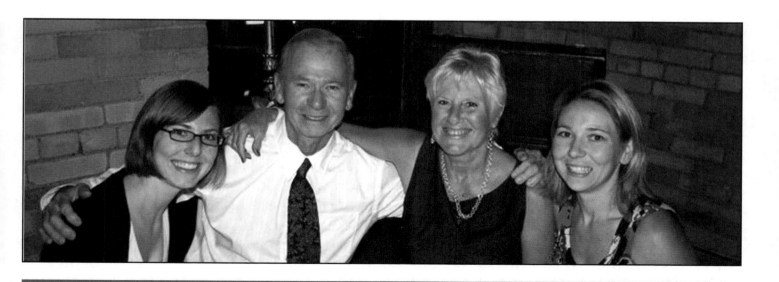

OUR LATEST FAMILY PHOTO

KNOCKED DOWN, BUT NOT OUT

The recession of 1991-1992 hit hard and our business revenues plummeted like a stone. We were caught in the perfect storm. We had just expanded our rental truck fleet (our core business), put on a huge building addition, and got back into the leasing business that provided zero cash flow for at least three years from the starting point in 1991. We racked up large losses and the banks panicked, pulling every penny of our line of credit. The line of credit went from $750,000.00 to 0 in less than 90 days, even after a 35-year relationship between the bank and my business partner. We scrambled and reduced our fleet by 50%, but in the end the vehicle finance company took back the remaining fleet and we were rendered insolvent on Friday, March 13, 1992. How prophetic is that - Friday the 13th! My 17 years of hard work, including many long nights and weekends, vanished before my eyes. To make matters worse, we had leveraged our family home to gain equity in the company and so we ended up losing the family home as well. We had to sell our family home and move into a rental home. Once again, life had thrown me another big surprise and this one was devastating. Within two months of losing the company and my home, I lost two good friends. Bill Harmatuk was a fellow employee I had known for over 15 years. He had a massive heart attack, likely precipitated by the events of 1992 when he was forced to find another job. Another friend, Marty Scheutjens, died of terminal brain cancer. All those events drove me deeper in the ditch. I managed to get the company restructured under new ownership, but I would never again be an owner of the business I had helped to build. I recall heading to work one cold rainy spring morning after the company restructuring, the death of my friends, and the move into a rental home. I was really down in the dumps. I saw a sight that changed my life forever. I witnessed a blind and crippled man struggling to walk down the street. It was at that moment I realized I had nothing to complain about, and that I had my health and my family. It was time for me to make a permanent change in my lifestyle.

REBUILDING

During the fall of the business I met a man who is now my best friend, Tony Cipollone. I formed a new company that dealt in buying and selling vehicles that was to be operated by Tony full time and myself on a part time basis. We could get no line of credit from any bank, but my mother in law lent us $30,000.00 at 15 % interest - a ridiculously high rate (done at my insistence) so that it greatly exceeded her return compared to other investments. Tony was incredible. We would be selling almost 30 used cars a month, but with very small margins. Tony would get the lion's share of the profit, which was not a lot, but it allowed him to pay his bills and we were able to accumulate enough to get my family and I back into a home. I am forever grateful to Tony for all he was able to do for us and for his loyalty when we were down on our luck. Tony went on to start his own business and has made a success of that. He also battled cancer, which involved a 12 hour throat cancer operation as a part of his treatment. I am happy to report that he has been in remission for over 10 years. I wish him and his wife Lucy good health and long lives.

I began training at the gym and completely changed my nutrition habits. I would put in a good 8 hours a week of hard work at the gym and spent countless hours researching nutrition and training information. I received some very good training techniques from other people at the gym who, in many cases, had been weight training for years. Unlike most others at the gym, I made sure that stretching, abdominals and a 30 minute cardio routine were a part of each and every workout in addition to weight training. I knew that in order to have "the whole package" (flexibility, power and endurance), I had to complete all four routines each day I trained. Before I started exercising, my waist had ballooned to almost 37 inches from 32 and my weight had climbed by 25lbs. I felt lazy and lethargic. But within a few months, I began to lose weight and gained a new sense of self worth and strength. My experience has shown that starting a fitness routine later in life does not limit what you can accomplish. I felt renewed and I was happy to be back in a home that we owned rather than rented.

During my "rebuilding phase," as I would describe it, I experienced another traumatic experience. My first motorcycle was a 1985 Yamaha V Max which, in its day, was the fastest production motorcycle in the world. Being speed crazy doesn't end at 40! I would only drive the bike a few times a year and I avoided city and highway traffic like the plague because I had heard too many horror stories of bad motorcycle accidents where vehicles do not see the motorcyclist. However, a gym member asked me to bring in my bike for him to see and during the trip into the city, a van cut right in front of me with no warning. I had a millisecond to react and avoid going directly into the side of the van, so I braked hard and swung to the curb. The bike hit the curb and flipped sideways in the air and landed squarely on my leg and elbow. I bounced down the road after the initial fall and

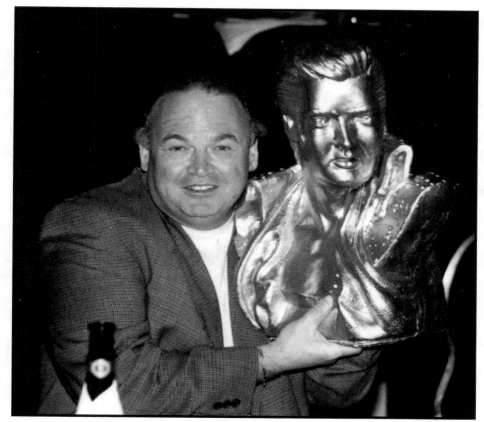

MY BEST FRIEND TONY WITH HIS IDOL ELVIS

was left with a smashed left elbow – that was fortunately not broken - and a blown main artery in my leg. Pavement is not very forgiving. I was in a lot of pain for a long time, but fortunately no surgery was required for the artery. The rest of my body did not show any signs of trauma despite the fall. I am confident that my fitness level had contributed to my survival and my recovery. Once again, I had dodged a bullet but I was fortunate that my injuries were not more severe, and I refused to let the accident end my commitment to fitness.

I began to get more and more frustrated at work with the owner of the business, and in the words of my physician, I was like "a pot of boiling water with a lid ready to explode". I could barely contain my rage and it was time to do something to take out my frustrations. I would take great pains to avoid losing my temper at home. Having a peaceful and harmonious home was a top priority for me. The solution: take up boxing at age 57 and continue my usual training, but at a much less rigorous pace. My body could not handle 12 hours of hard exercise each week in addition to running a business. I needed to get occasional massages to take out the knotted muscles from such intense training. While it is important to push yourself in your fitness routines, it is equally important not to overdo it.

Within three months of beginning boxing, I shed another 14 lbs on my small frame. I got down to 159 lbs which was only 2 lbs more than I weighed 25 years before. My boxing training consisted of 1 hour sessions 3 times a week with two former lightweight champions of Canada and another world class trainer. Most of the time it was one-on-one training for one hour, pretty well at a non-stop pace. I knew I was fit before I began boxing, but I really did not expect boxing to be as difficult as it was. Let me tell you - when you think you are in great shape, put on a pair of 14 ounce gloves and spar for three rounds with an experienced fighter who challenges you. You will get a whole new respect for what boxers have to endure. I gained the respect of the members of the boxing club and went on to weight train the eight time national Canadian lightweight amateur champion Ibrahim Kamal for seven weeks. He did not put on a pound of weight during the training, but he certainly gained a lot of power during that short stint. I know that I won over his respect with my knowledge and experience when he realized what power gains he made and when he saw what I could do in the gym.

While boxing is not necessarily an   appropriate choice for everyone, I think it's important to consider options when it comes to your health and fitness. While the majority of this book is focused on gym routines, you can obviously expand your fitness routine to include other activities that you find enjoyable.

TURNING 60 — LET'S PARTY!

The age of 60 was a milestone for me and I wanted to do something special, so I invited a large number of my favorite ladies that I had met during the course of my life to my 60th birthday party. I would do all the cooking and they would enjoy the results. A total of 14 ladies, and of course my wife and daughters, attended the birthday party at our home. It was a fabulous party – lots of laughter, a selection of fine wines, and plenty of good food. In addition to a huge assortment of appetizers, I served my homemade "deadly" Caesar salad, my homemade squash soup and a homemade seafood soup. For the main course, we had veal tenderloin, pork tenderloin and lamb tenderloin along

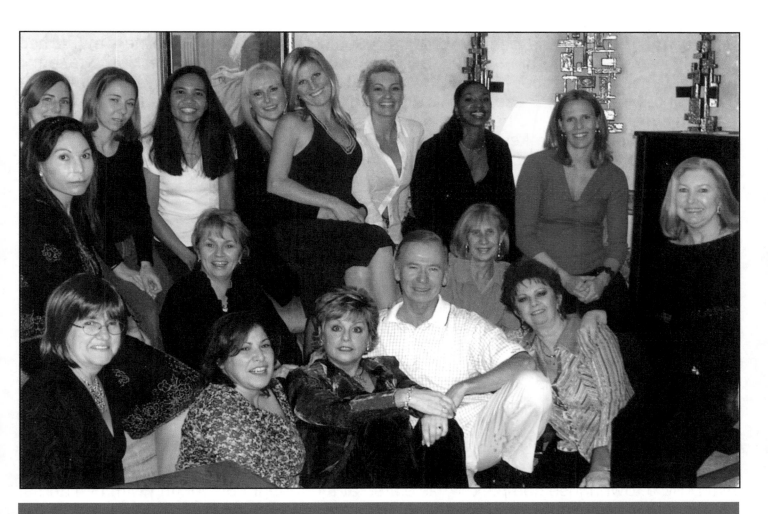

COOKING FOR 17 LADIES - A VERY HECTIC EVENING PREPARING THE MEALS, BUT ONE ENJOYED BY ALL - FINE FOOD, GREAT WINES, AND LOTS OF LAUGHTER

with a multitude of steamed fresh vegetables. It truly was a memorable evening, and one that I will remember with great fondness forever.

NEW DIRECTIONS

The relationship between the owner of the business and myself continued to be a source of great irritation to me. But I was fortunately surrounded by a wonderful group of loyal and competent staff, many of whom had been working with me for almost 30 years. It was like a family - everyone got along well and worked together like a well oiled machine. These staff members are what kept me at the company. In 2004, we received an opportunity to add a world class Japanese truck franchise to the existing business, and I spent a year of hard work putting together the business plan to acquire the franchise. Within two months of acquiring the franchise, the owner walked in the door and announced that his nephew was joining the company to run the new truck franchise. I was beside myself with anger. I was President and General Manager of the entire operation, and he did not have the common decency or wisdom to discuss his nephew's hiring with the person who was running his business. The nephew turned out to be arrogant and shortsighted, and the owner and his nephew set out to take the company in a new direction. I knew it was time to leave and so I gave my notice. It was a very painful decision because I was so attached to the people I had been working with for so many years. Within two business days of my leaving, the owner abruptly terminated the employment of two key administrative employees who, under my authority, had been hardworking, loyal, and competent, for over 30 years, and began to overhaul the entire operation. Within two years of my leaving, the company added managers and administration staff in numbers that far exceeded what was necessary for the business, filed for bankruptcy protection, and the nephew eventually left the company. Almost all the original staff either resigned or were terminated. All in all, not a happy ending for anyone.

I was a little like a rudderless ship for a few months, not knowing what course to pursue. In the end, I made very poor career choices that only brought more frustration. My family and I were also dealing with moving homes during this time and a mother-in-law with advanced Alzheimer's disease. I had moved my wife out of Toronto to the small village of Bloomfield, Ontario, to at least put her in a position of less stress. I had taken a position in Toronto that was clearly not a right fit and so I gave my notice to the new employer and moved to Bloomfield to be with my wife full time. I was not sure what to do at this point and I felt frustrated, helpless, hopeless, and depressed. Nothing seemed to be going right.

Then my brother, sensing my frustration, offered to have me come to Saskatoon to help him build a townhouse complex. I was elated at the thought of working with him and at least being somewhat in control of my own destiny. We were only three weeks into the job when an accident took place. We were working seven days a week for long hours and late in the day, when I would start to get tired, it was difficult to be as attentive as I was in earlier hours. I had not covered the holes for the staircases on the main floor and in the process of setting up a dividing wall on the main floor, I had stepped backward into one of the holes and fell into the basement onto gravel. It all happened in a split second, which shocked my brother and his other helper. There was no opportunity for them to react before I fell. The fall resulted in three fractured vertebrae, a concussion, and a badly bruised kneecap that had caught the edge of the main floor during the fall. But as the saying goes, "all's well that ends well". That certainly applies in my case and this book is the result of that incident. It was my brother who suggested during my recuperation that I should think about what to do after I had recovered and to consider something that I did well and enjoyed. Fitness training and nutrition came to mind, and I can only hope that my experience and enjoyment of fitness comes through this book and can assist you in the betterment of your own health and fitness.

REMAINING LUCK

My wife and I headed to Florida in December 2010, when I was in the process of writing this book. On the trip down, I had another episode take place that could have resulted in my demise. We had been driving for three days and about 20 minutes from our final destination, off Interstate I-95, I heard a loud thumping from the front end of our van. The traffic was going at least 120 kms per hour and was solid throughout the highway, but I knew it sounded serious so I slowed to about 80 kms per hour and limped in to Melbourne, Florida. The next day, I took the van to a local garage to discover that all the wheel nuts on the front left wheel were loose to the point that you could turn them with your fingers. In addition to the loose wheel nuts, two of the studs that hold the nuts had sheared off completely. We should have lost a front wheel on I-95 at high speed, in busy traffic. Had that taken place, it would have likely resulted in a catastrophe.

I have had a lot of good luck and a lot of bad luck in my life. But I am lucky to be alive given the number and the severity of some of the incidents that took place. The one thing in my life that I do not need any more of is big surprises. I look forward to a slower paced life focused on health and happiness, and I hope I can pass that focus on to my friends, family, and even to you.

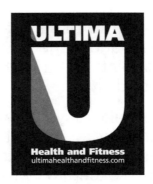

CHAPTER
2

THE FIVE KEYS TO FITNESS

In my view, there are five keys to fitness and health, each of which is important to master in order to achieve your goals of good health and fitness. I believe that you need to follow all of these basic principles to reach your full potential. They are as follows:

1. **Patience**

2. **Consistency**

3. **Hard work**

4. **A good training program**

5. **Proper nutrition**

1. PATIENCE
We live in a world where clever marketing techniques try to make people believe that there is always a short cut to achieving their goals. It may be in the form of a pill, or some quick and easy exercise program, or a "new and improved" machine or piece of fitness equipment. The claim is made that they are going to magically change your body in a matter of days or weeks, and with very little effort. The truth is that most of these programs are doomed to fail because they rarely produce the benefits they promise,

especially when it comes to long-term or lasting effects. When one fails to see the results that these quick fixes promise, and in the time frame that they claim, it is easy to see why so many people feel disappointment and defeat. So you give up, and then try another routine, and that also fails to deliver.

Proper health and fitness does not take days or weeks to achieve. It takes months and years of work to achieve. So instead of trying the latest quick fix, you need to be committed to a change in your lifestyle, and it will take patience and time. Remember that good things take time, and it is no exception when it comes to making a permanent change to your body.

2. CONSISTENCY

I cannot overemphasize the importance of consistency. Working at an exercise routine like a mad fiend for several days or weeks, or going on some extreme diet for a short period of time and then suddenly stopping, thinking that you can get back to where you left off, does not work. Once again, it takes months and years of consistent behavior, to positively improve and reshape your body and your life. So set yourself both training goals and nutritional goals after you have read this book and make sure that your efforts remain consistent over time to reach these goals. Let nothing stand in your way to reach the finish line. Make health and fitness your most consistent discipline and let family and health be your first priority. Everything else takes a second seat.

3. HARD WORK

I cannot overstate the number of years I watched people spend an hour or more on a cardio machine (or on training of any kind) and never break a sweat. You need to constantly - but gently, and slowly - raise the performance bar as time goes on. Gradually increase the intensity of your efforts until you see and feel the results of increased performance. You will be amazed at what you can achieve with time and effort. The latter chapters will provide guidance in this area, outlining a progression in fitness levels one can achieve, including instruction for the duration of routines, the number of training routines in a week, and how to target specific body parts. A fitness routine that challenges you and encourages you to work hard will be a positive, rewarding experience when you achieve your fitness goals.

4. A GOOD TRAINING PROGRAM

If you do not have a good training program, you will not achieve the results you should be reaching. This book is an excellent basis for your training and is based on my 18 years of fitness training, including over 8,000 hours in the gym and countless hours researching training methods and techniques. After you have read the book in full and tested the training methods, you may want to get a good personal trainer to help you get started or get motivated. Choose a trainer who comes highly recommended by friends or associates. Your trainer should have a proven and verifiable track record of success with clients. If your trainer is pushing you to total exhaustion early on in the training, get another trainer. The old adage "walk before you run" holds true in developing a long term training plan. Within three months of training with a professional, you may be capable of developing and performing your own program, using this book as your guide. However it is important to remember that everyone has a different learning curve and you should be comfortable with a training plan that works best for you. You may also want to keep notes on each training routine to keep track of your progress, especially in your first few months of training. I have seen others who keep notes for years. Again, do what works best for you.

A good training partner can also help in your development. Beginning as a motivator and as a friend, a training partner can be mutually beneficial as you both learn to build on your fitness training. As you both develop your fitness and health, you should begin to challenge yourself and your partner as you increase the intensity of your training. Finally, a training partner can be a great help in spotting you once you begin to lift heavier weights. A later chapter will deal with the importance of a good spotter to avoid injury and to help you increase your repetitions on each exercise.

The ultimate goal should be a proper lean weight for your body frame, together with the three most important basics of flexibility, power, and endurance. Please do not concentrate on one item, such as power. I have seen many people who are extremely powerful but have no flexibility, or are helpless on abdominal routines and can last no more than five minutes on a difficult 30 minute cardio routine. A fit, lean, and athletic body is best for long term health.

5. PROPER NUTRITION

If you do not eat properly, you will not achieve proper health and fitness. Food is one of the building blocks of your body, and you must eat the right foods - in proper and reasonable quantities - to ensure the best long term results. Good quality water is another crucial element for the proper long term development of your body and health. A later chapter deals with this important issue. Vitamin and mineral supplements are also essential to you, and again, a later chapter deals with this subject.

I do not recommend eating out at restaurants - especially fast food chains - as the main source for your nutrition. In most cases, we have no idea how much salt, calories, saturated fats, or trans fats these establishments have in their food. In many instances, the food served is not balanced nutritionally and is detrimental for your long term health if consumed on a regular basis. The occasional meal at a restaurant or fast food establishment will not be too harmful, but it is unwise to make it your regular source for food. Again, later chapters will provide guidance for selecting foods that are much healthier for you.

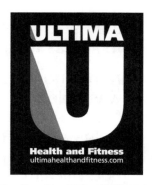

CHAPTER
3

THE HEALTH BENEFITS OF REGULAR EXERCISE

There is plenty of good evidence to support the principle that exercise plays a significant role in the betterment of your long-term health. The world famous Mayo Clinic names the following benefits of regular exercise:

1. **It improves your mood, likely reducing depression and anxiety, so you are able to better handle stressful situations**

2. **It combats chronic diseases**

3. **It helps you manage your weight**

4. **It boosts your energy level**

5. **It promotes sleep**

6. **It can put the spark back in your sex life**

Daily physical activity can help prevent heart disease and stroke by lowering blood pressure, improving your high-density lipoprotein (HDL) good cholesterol and reducing your low-density lipoprotein (LDL) bad cholesterol. It can also aid in the control of non insulin-dependent diabetes by reducing body fat. Physical activity increases muscle strength and endurance, improves flexibility, and helps to prevent joint pain. Weight bearing exercises promote bone density to help stave off osteoporosis. The list of benefits is almost endless and if you feel so inclined, you can research the benefits of fitness online or in your public library to see countless more. In simple terms, there are just too many benefits to ignore. For the betterment of your own health and wellbeing, you need to get active with an effective fitness routine and the sooner, the better.

Once I began my own exercise program, I noticed an immediate improvement in my own self-esteem and mental focus. I was able to gain increased strength and stamina, while at the same time losing body fat and building muscle. I am confident that anyone can get the same results as I did with the right attitude and perseverance. However, the first few weeks of training are taxing. You may feel sore and tired, but please stick with the program. After a few weeks, you will almost certainly begin to feel and see the results. I believe that the choice to make this change in your lifestyle is something you will not regret, and it will become a good "habit" as the years go by.

CHOOSING A PROPER EXERCISE PROGRAM

There are a vast array of exercise programs to choose from that are effective. This book focuses on a program that can be used as a launching pad for you to pursue other exercises that may be more appealing to you once you achieve the goals of proper bodyweight, flexibility, strength and endurance. Once you make a commitment to start anew and begin to train, you may find that a number of other activities may be used to supplement this program. But remember to get in good physical condition before you begin competitive sports – do not use competitive sports to get in good physical condition. Injuries sustained in competitive sports often take place when you place too much stress on a body that is not properly prepared for that stress.

In place of my suggested stretching exercises, you may find that Yoga, Pilates, or the Swiss Ball is a better substitute. The most important thing is that you set out to accomplish your essential stretching routines by one of these methods.

Skipping, swimming, running, hiking, walking, cycling, boxing, and tennis are just some of the aerobic exercises designed to focus on cardiovascular endurance and could be used in place of my suggested cardio routines. Choose the one that you enjoy the most.

Abdominals and your lower back should be worked on regularly and properly to ensure that you have good core strength to support your entire upper body, to provide good posture, and to prevent back pain or back injuries. Many of the exercises demonstrated in this book are utilized for obtaining a strong core. You may want to add Bosu ball exercises for additional work to the stabilizer muscles.

I firmly believe that there are tremendous benefits to weight training that can be achieved by anyone, regardless of age. Do not feel the least bit intimidated by weight training or the gym environment because the betterment of your health and fitness is not a competition with those around you, it is an accomplishment that is highly personalized for you alone. If you simply follow the demonstrations of the training exercises in this book, you should be able to train injury free and gradually see your body reshape and strengthen dramatically.

The overriding principal in choosing a healthier lifestyle is that you must start a program and follow through. There is no benefit to quitting after a short stint. You must be mentally committed to making a permanent change in your lifestyle. It does not matter what age or weight you begin your training with. Once you get started with a routine and begin to maintain new control over your life, I am confident that you will be motivated to look to the future instead of falling back into old habits. If you work hard, persevere through your times of low motivation, and refuse to give up, you may be surprised at how dramatic the changes in your health can be. Good luck and best wishes in your pursuit of a new you.

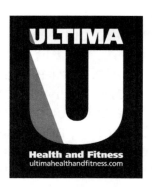

CHAPTER
4

OBESITY AND DIABETES EPIDEMICS
IN THE WESTERN WORLD

There are literally mountains of written data and other scientific evidence to support the argument that the world—and North America in particular—is having an epidemic of obesity that all too often results in diabetes. The World Health Organization (WHO), a globally recognized and reputable source of information, presents a vast array of maps, tables and statistics showing the extent of the obesity problem on their website (www.who.int). Their obesity map of North America shows that 23.1 % of adult Canadians and 33.9% of adult Americans are classified as obese. The Federal Government of Canada also released a study on obesity that was published on July 15, 2005, through the Library of Parliament titled "The Obesity Epidemic in Canada". The Centre for Disease Control and Prevention (CDC) in the United States, a leading health agency in the U.S., reported in 2009 that there had been a significant increase in obesity in the U.S., notably during the last 20 years.

Obesity can also lead to diabetes. The WHO reports on their website that diabetes has increasingly become a global problem that can be linked to inactivity and obesity. They go on to predict that the number of deaths from diabetes will double between 2005 and 2030. The U.S. Department of Health and Human Services reported in 2008 that diabetes was the 7th leading cause of death. Given that obesity is a main cause of diabetes, it is not a far stretch to make the claim that obesity itself is a leading cause of death. I know first hand what diabetes can do to one's body. My sister-in-law Marlene had Type 1 diabetes from the age of four. She ended up with a quadruple heart bypass, total blindness, three amputations, and a heart attack that resulted in her death. Diabetes is a relentless disease that holds no mercy for anyone that it strikes.

Obesity and resulting diabetes is costing our North American health care systems well in excess of one hundred billion dollars. In the U.S. alone, the cost of healthcare for the year 2003 was seventy-five billion dollars (as stated by the U.S. Centre for Disease Control) and the cost is growing exponentially as the situation worsens. Just imagine what the costs will amount to in 20 years if our communities don't start making lifestyle changes. The numbers would be staggering and obesity (and resulting diabetes) would likely be one of the major health costs in the future. An increased focus on treating obese and diabetic patients may also lead to reductions in other critical care issues.

Because of the proven problems obesity can cause, there is essentially universal acceptance by leading authorities that we have a serious problem to address. While some obesity can be attributed to genetics, most obesity can be linked back to three simple facts:

1. We eat too much

2. We eat the wrong foods

3. We do not exercise enough

Therefore, most cases of obesity are preventable and I believe the epidemic can be remedied with simple changes throughout our communities. First, I believe we need national programs spearheaded by federal and provincial (or state) governments that initiate mandatory nutrition and physical education programs in elementary and high schools. The health of our children should be the biggest priority for the education system, yet I believe it has not been appropriately responded to because of the perpetual rise in obesity and inactivity in children and teens. Let's be practical and use common sense in addressing the obesity problem. Establishing good nutrition and exercise is essential to the long term health of our children. The existing system unfortunately does not seem to recognize and address the obesity problem as it should. The education system, as it now stands, is primarily designed to provide skills and knowledge for students to make their way into the work force. While these types of courses are mandatory, courses on health and nutrition—as well as courses that provide increased physical activity—often remain optional and are therefore phased out of the majority of students' schedules. Health and wellbeing have to stop being so easily passed by for young students.

We need to change the mindset of the bureaucrats who administer our education system and put in place the necessary changes to education that will provide future generations with the basic tools to ensure good health. We also need the general public to be aware of the problem and practical and easily understandable solutions should be presented through various media outlets including television, the Internet, newspapers, radio, and so forth.

Chapters 5 through 20 deal with proper nutrition and exercise programs. These chapters will provide you with essential information to avoid becoming a statistic in the growing obesity epidemic.

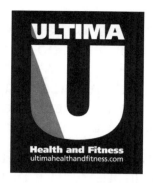

CHAPTER
5

WATER—THE MOST IMPORTANT INGREDIENT THAT YOU PUT IN YOUR BODY

Since more than 50% of your body - including your bones, your muscles, your blood and even your brain - is made up of water, it only makes common sense that you should be drinking good quality water. Quality water helps to ensure that your body is getting the very best that it needs to function in a healthy manner for the long term.

The water from your taps is likely being treated by local authorities to the best of their abilities, given massive volume requirements of cities and limited financial budgets. Because of these restraints things like chlorine, a known carcinogen, can be used to purify the water. Unfortunately, authorities are unable to remove a vast array of other toxic chemicals such as pesticides, metals, industrial chemicals, and insecticides. Lead piping was used almost exclusively to supply water to homes and businesses prior to 1961. Furthermore, leads and lead solder was used on water pipes for most houses built before 1987. Lead is a highly toxic substance that is dangerous to your health, even at low levels. In 2010, the Environmental Working Group in the U.S.A. studied the drinking water in 35 American cities and found chromium-6 in 31 of the 35 cities sampled. Chromium-6 is recognized as a human carcinogen. The Environmental Working Group also undertook a five year study ending in 2009 studying the quality of water in most major U.S. cities. The five year study is important because it shows the persistent presence of chemicals in drinking water. Test results from the national database reported a total of 316 contaminants in water supplied to 256 million Americans in 48,000 communities, and that among the contaminants, there were 202 chemicals that are not subject to any government regulation or safety standards for drinking water. Perchlorates used in rocket fuel have been discovered in 2010 in the drinking water of

86 water systems in California. Babies who drank water even slightly contaminated by perchlorate had a 50% chance of developing poorly performing thyroid glands according to Dr. Craig Steinmaus, lead author of the study. In reading these studies it becomes evident that there are many toxins and chemicals that are often not removed and have to be processed by your body, which will likely affect your long term health. In short, tap water is a poor first choice for your body's needs and for your long term well-being.

As a response to the general mistrust of the safety of tap water, bottled water has developed into a multi billion dollar industry. But bottled water may still have the same problems that remain with tap water. Companies that sell bottled waters offer a whole range of products, including carbonated water, tap water, well water, glacier water, distilled water, and even rain water. In short, there is no consistency in knowing what you are actually drinking. To top it off, we are creating a huge environmental problem with billions of plastic bottles being sold that may or may not be recycled. Lastly, bottled water is expensive – not only for the consumer but also for cities to process both garbage and recycling.

Some individuals swear by the purity of well water, but that too has its drawbacks. Well water can be easily contaminated by herbicides, pesticides and animal waste that leach into the underground streams that feed the wells over time. And gas and oil fraccing has caused many wells to be so badly contaminated that they can not be used for human or animal consumption. To see clear proof of such contamination, I highly recommend watching the documentary "GasLand" (Dir. Josh Fox, 2010). If you decide to continue using well water, then at the very least get your water tested by a reputable independent laboratory every three months to ensure that the water you are ingesting is relatively clean.

But let's look at a very simple solution that eliminates any guesswork.

Distilled water is as pure as you can get, and you can buy machines that can produce several liters of unquestionably pure water each day. Distilled water machines provide a long lasting solution - one of my best friends and his wife have been using distilled water systems for over 30 years. They use two units in their household for all their needs, and the maintenance on the units is minimal. Distilled water systems should be your first choice in obtaining quality water.

Personally, I have been using a reverse osmosis system for over 25 years to get clean water. It is one step down from distilled water, but is slightly more convenient in terms of maintenance and greater water production. It uses a simple separate faucet on your sink which is connected to a series of filters and a storage canister. You will need to change annually: a pre-filter, a post-filter, and a carbon filter. Then every two years or so, you will likely need to change the membrane filter that removes the finest of impurities. Your supplier should provide you with test kits to be mailed for testing every six months to ensure you are getting maximum quality and to let you know when filters need to be changed.

Next, you need to decide what container to use to store your water. Plastic is easily contaminated, and glass – though technically a reliable choice - is heavy, awkward, and prone to breakage. I recommend purchasing two or three stainless steel containers that can be sanitized in a dishwasher so that you always have a clean one on hand. Make sure that the container holds at least two liters of water so that you do not have to constantly refill from another source.

In choosing a distilled water system or reverse osmosis system, individuals can make a notable difference in reducing bottle waste and can save hundreds of dollars in the long run. Make the right healthy choice, and the right financial decision, by producing your own pure water that you know is best for you.

You should consume at least two to three liters of clean water each day. During my two-hour workouts I consume about two litres of water. I complete these workouts four days a week. I constantly sip water between each training routine, and also during my 30 minute cardio routine. It takes a few weeks for your body to get used to ingesting these quantities, but stick with the plan. Your body will thank you as you begin a new exercise program and as your body ages. It needs to be constantly rehydrated to remain healthy, strong and vibrant.

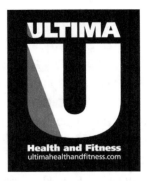

CHAPTER
6

WEIGHT LOSS AND PROPER NUTRITION WITH FOOD PLANS

There are literally thousands of weight loss plans available, many of them promising quick and easy results in as little as a few days. Companies spend millions of dollars on advertising and marketing programs trying to convince you that they have the one diet that will work. They may provide extreme examples of success stories where some clients lose as much as 30 pounds or more in as little as 30 days. You should note however, that almost all of these diet plans never even mention exercise as part of a successful result, which is an enormous mistake in my view. Quick, easy, painless, fat release and fat burning is the mantra of most of these commercially advertised diets. It sounds so simple - too bad so many of these diets end up as failure. All too often their clients continue to struggle with weight problems and spend vast amounts of money with little or no progress or they revert back to their old weight after temporary improvement.

This book is dedicated to providing you with a realistic, sensible, and long term solution to weight control issues. What you need is a rational and proven food plan that focuses on the quality of food in proper portions rather than some quick fix diet. I hope to present realistic alternatives that leave you feeling satisfied with meals providing proper nutrition, variety and good taste. You also must make the effort to exercise in order to burn off excess fat. The process will take longer than the usual commercial diets being offered but the results will last a lifetime if you persevere and stick with the game plan. If you suffer from binge eating, or another eating disorder, you need to receive professional help before you begin this program.

It's necessary to start with a few basic principles that need to be followed like any other daily ritual that you perform. The principles listed on the next page need to be photocopied and posted on your refrigerator and read daily as a constant reminder of what you need to do to reach your goals. Every time you open the fridge, "the list" will be there to remind you to make the right choices. You need to faithfully follow the principles on "the list" until they are ingrained in your mind for life. Try your very best to come as close as you possibly can to all the principles outlined on "the list". I know how difficult it is to be disciplined in your eating habits. The first few weeks are the hardest to get through. However, once you begin to see the beneficial results that the list provides, you will never return to your old bad habits. You must think of these rules as your means to achieve proper nutrition and weight control. Within three months, I am confident that you will start to see the benefits of following this course that cannot be achieved with other commercial diet plans.

THE LIST

1. Drink 2 to 3 litres of clean water as outlined in Chapter 5
2. No snacks between meals or after your last meal of the day
3. Eat no white carbohydrates – no white bread, no white rice, no white potatoes. Substitute whole grain breads, brown rice and sweet potato as healthier alternatives.
4. Try to split lunch into two meals – one late morning and one mid-afternoon
5. You must exercise at least four times per week for at least one hour each time. Use this book as your guide. If you are overweight or obese, use low impact, long duration cardio routines to burn fat
6. Do not use fast food restaurants as your regular source of food. Use the meals that are suggested in this book, which are far healthier
7. Read nutrition labels on food being purchased so that you know what your food contains in terms of fats and salts. Keep fat intake as close to zero as possible.
8. Your food choices should be as follows:
   ° First choice: certified Organic (if it is available and within your budget)
   ° Second choice: fresh foods
   ° Third choice: frozen foods (including frozen vegetables)
   ° Last choice: canned goods (too much salt and preservatives)
9. Reduce your salt intake as much as possible. The meal plans photographed and described in this book are low in salt
10. Choose low glycemic foods. Please see http://www.fifty50.com for glycemic index for all food groups. Also choose low acidic foods. Most of the food choices in the daily menus in this book are low glycemic and low acidic
11. Eliminate trans fats and saturated fats whenever possible from your food supply. Refer to item # 7 to determine fat content when purchasing products
12. Trim all fat from meats being prepared.
13. Cook with extra virgin olive oil or canola oil in place of saturated fat such as butter
14. Steam all your vegetables whenever possible
15. Do not smoke cigarettes
16. Do not use illicit drugs
17. Limit your alcohol intake to once per week in moderate amounts

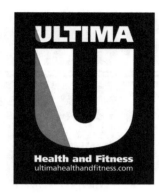

Meal Plan for Healthy Nutrition and Weight Control*

* Important Note:
It will take you about three weeks to get used to the change in your diet but I am confident that you will begin to enjoy the different tastes of the meals, as well as see the positive results to your body. Please do not give up on these meals and depend on fast food establishments – persevere and you will reap the rewards.

BREAKFAST

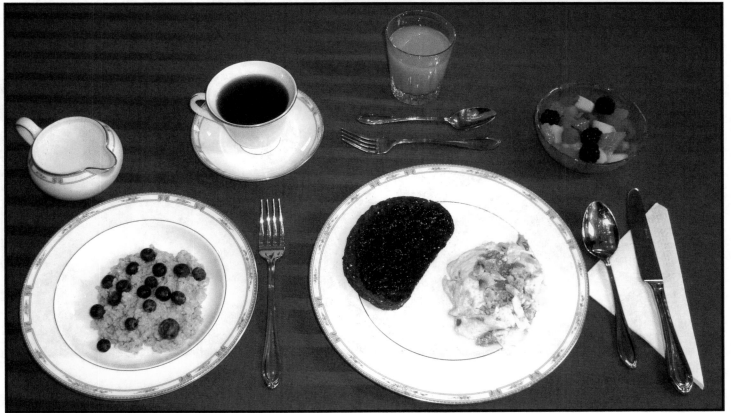

1. One glass of tangerine juice with one teaspoon of organic flax oil mixed in - this will meet your omega 3 and omega 6 essential fatty acid needs for the day.

2. One medium bowl of fruit containing any or all of the following: grapefruit, strawberries, raspberries, blackberries, orange slices, pineapple, melon – including watermelon and cantaloupe.

3. One medium bowl of non-instant oatmeal or high fibre/low sugar cereal. Blueberries may be added for flavour. Do not add any sugar. Use a little skim milk.

4. Fried egg whites only (no yolk) cooked in a touch of extra virgin olive oil instead of butter. Add a little ketchup or salsa for flavour. Egg white omelettes may be substituted for fried egg whites and can include mushroom, tomato, peppers, and onions.

5. One or two slices of pumpernickel bread with a thin spread of butter and sugar free jam. I recommend St. Dalfours sugar-free jam from France.

6. If you are in the habit of having coffee or tea, prepare it with milk instead of cream and minimal amounts of sugar.

LUNCH

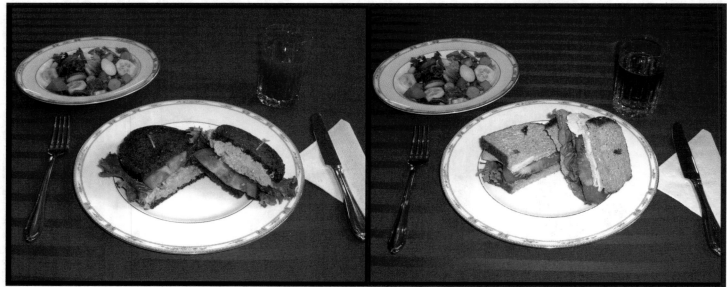

OPTION 1.   OPTION 2.

1. If you are able to, please split this meal into two small meals – the first in the late morning and the second in the mid-afternoon.

2. Garden salad with leaf lettuce, romaine, or spring mix. Add cucumber, celery, carrots, radishes, mushrooms, tomato, radicchio, peppers and other fresh vegetables to your liking. Prepare with an extra virgin olive oil and vinegar dressing, or a low fat dressing that you enjoy. You can make an extra large salad with these ingredients.

3. Any one of the following sandwiches made on pumpernickel bread: salmon, tuna, egg salad, or turkey. Use a little light mayonnaise to mix with salmon, tuna, or egg. Do not spread additional mayonnaise or butter to the bread. You can add lettuce and tomato and you can make an extra large sandwich.

    Large glass of low sodium tomato juice or vegetable cocktail, unsweetened apple juice, unsweetened cranberry juice or water.

DINNER

1. Salad as with lunch. Change the type daily for variety. Try garden, Caesar, spinach, spring mix and so forth.

2. a) Any ocean fish with optional shrimps, scallops and/or lobster. Poach or bake fish in lemon juice and water, with spices added to taste.

   b) Turkey, skinless chicken, pork tenderloin, veal, lean cuts of beef, lamb, venison, rabbit, or bison. When preparing meat, remove all fat. Please do not use butter to cook meats - use a little extra virgin olive oil in its place.

   c) Whole wheat pasta with a tomato sauce that is low in salt and sugar (see #7 on theList – always check the nutrition labels)

   d) You can choose to use the following vegetarian choices as a substitute for the proteins listed above: soybeans or soy flour, textured vegetable protein, tofu, seitan/wheat gluten (not for gluten intolerant people, or those who have celiac disease), or nuts (these are high in calories, so watch your intake).

   e) Many of the vegetables listed below can also help you meet your protein needs: Sweet potato, yam, brown rice, or wild rice.

3. Steamed or boiled broccoli, asparagus, cauliflower, green beans, kidney beans, beets, bok choy, snow peas, cabbage, brussels sprouts, turnip, leeks, onions, parsnips, peppers, spinach, or baked squash. Mushrooms can also be chosen and should be cooked in a little extra virgin olive oil. Occasional carrots, peas, or corn can be used for variety in taste.

4. For dessert, use fruits from breakfast. These fruits can also be substituted by a banana, apple, pear or other fruit you enjoy.

5. Large glass of water or sugar free juice.

When cooking your seafood, meats and vegetables, I recommend experimenting with different spices to get a greater variety of tastes. Make notes over time to see which spices you enjoy the most in each recipe. Just because these meals are healthy doesn't mean they can't taste great.

As mentioned in an earlier chapter, cooking has been a hobby of mine for over 20 years. I experimented with meals until I discovered what tasted the best and was healthy at the same time. I also experimented with a number of spices to see what seemed to go best with different meats and fish and sauces. Based on my experiences, I am recommending seven of my favourite dinners that I hope you enjoy.

DINNER: DAY 1

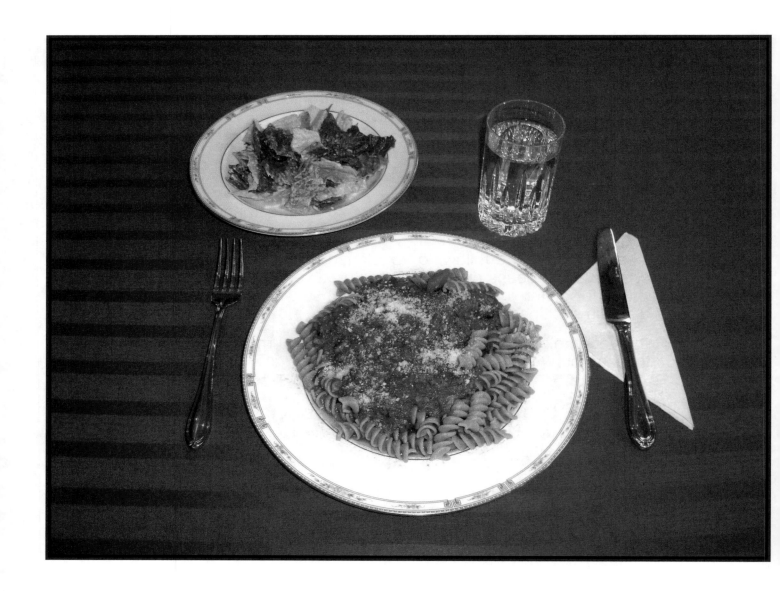

Whole wheat pasta with a tomato based sauce and extra lean ground beef, with the following spices or other items added for flavour: basil, bay leaves, fine herbs, oregano, Italian spices, chili peppers, fresh garlic, fine chop mushrooms, fine chop onions, sweet peppers, celery, and spinach. Experiment with small amounts of the spices first and then add more to taste as you cook. Top with light sprinkling of parmesan cheese.

Caesar salad prepared with fresh romaine lettuce, fresh lemon juice, light Caesar dressing.

Fresh fruit.

DINNER: DAY 2

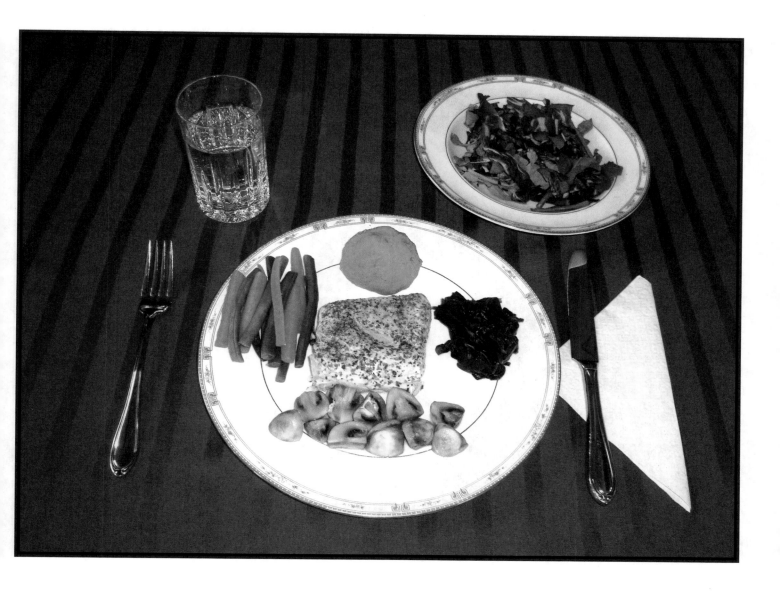

Salmon poached in mixture of water, a little dry white wine of your choice, and lemon juice with the following spices added for flavour: basil, cilantro, dill (very strong – go easy), fine herbs.

Steamed green beans, carrots and spinach.

Whipped sweet potato with a light sprinkling of low sodium salt and pepper.

Arugula and radicchio salad with balsamic vinaigrette

Fresh fruit.

DINNER: DAY 3

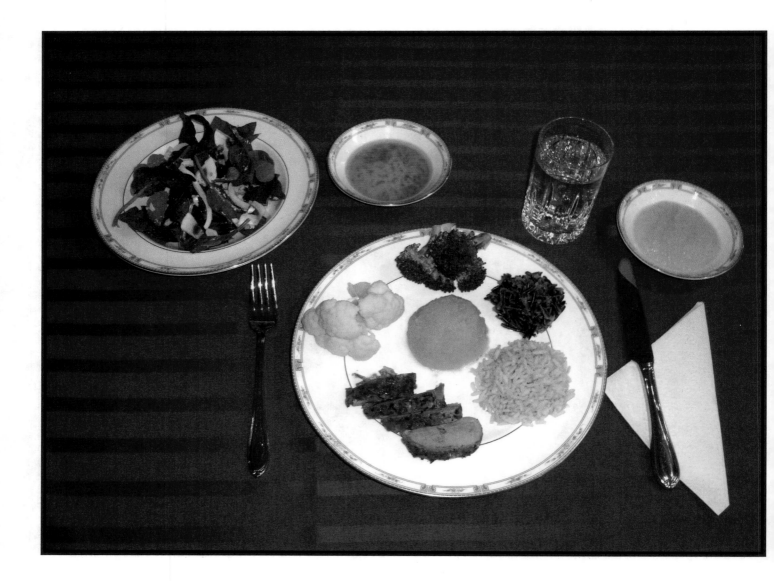

Pork tenderloin cooked with light coating of honey garlic sauce, drained can of mandarin oranges, pepper, fine herbs, marjoram, rosemary (go easy), thyme, summer savory. Bake in the oven at 350 degrees Fahrenheit for 45 minutes.

Steamed brown and wild rice in low sodium chicken stock.

Steamed cauliflower and broccoli and boiled turnip.

Unsweetened apple sauce.

Spinach salad (See recipe on next page)

Fresh fruit

MARLENE MURRAY'S SPINACH SALAD

As I mentioned earlier in chapter 4, my sister in law fought her entire lifetime against the ravages of type 1 diabetes. This recipe was one of her favourites, and it is an honour to share it with you.

Ingredients:
- 1 package of fresh spinach
- 4 eggs – hard-boiled, sliced
- 1/4 cup sliced almonds
- Fresh mushrooms and/or mandarins and parmesan cheese to taste

Dressing:
- 2/3 cup olive oil
- 2 cloves of garlic, crushed
- 1/4 cup of wine vinegar
- 1 tsp. tarragon
- 1 tsp. salt
- 1/4 tsp. pepper
- pinch of dry mustard

DINNER: DAY 4

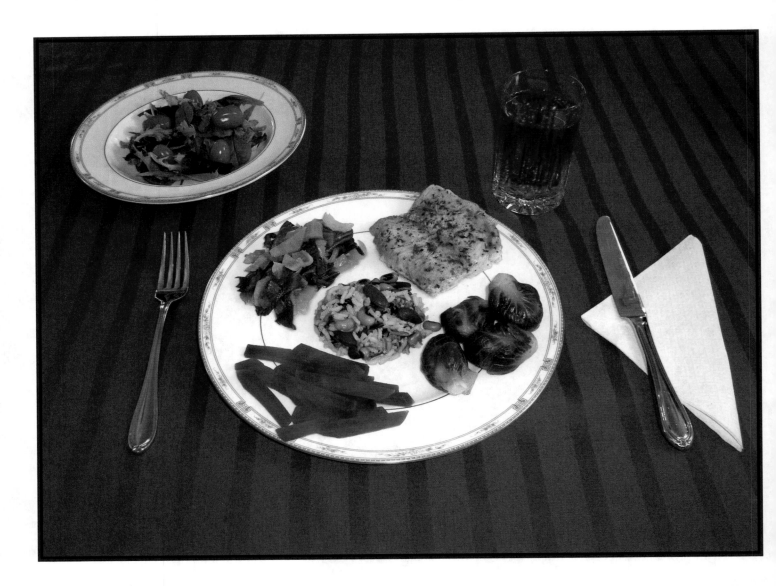

Skinless chicken breast with light coating of honey garlic sauce, pepper, fine herbs, marjoram, rosemary (go easy), sage (go very easy), thyme. Rabbit can be substituted for chicken with the same spices. Add a little water to the saucepan.

Or, if you like something more spicy :

Skinless chicken breast marinated overnight with mushroom soya sauce, then before cooking, put on a light coating of Jamaican jerk sauce, fine herbs, thyme. Cook for 30 minutes on low heat on the stovetop, turning occasionally.

Steamed brown rice and wild rice in low sodium chicken stock, boiled kidney beans and black eyed peas, brussels sprouts, bok choy, beets.

Garden salad with extra virgin olive oil and vinegar.

Fresh fruit.

DINNER: DAY 5

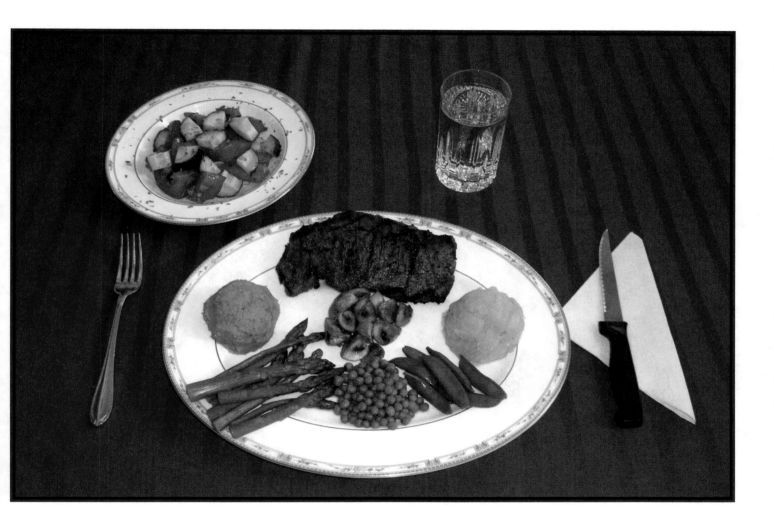

Strip loin steak with all fat trimmed, lightly seasoned with garlic salt and pepper.

Or: Beef or veal tenderloin (somewhat costly) with light sprinkling of garlic salt, pepper, fine herbs, marjoram, summer savory, rosemary, thyme.

Or: Venison or Bison with same spices as tenderloin above.

Or: Lamb with all fat trimmed with dijon mustard or mint sauce for flavour.

BBQ steak.

Whipped sweet potatoes – no salt but add a little pepper.

Steamed asparagus, baked squash, peas, mushrooms cooked in extra virgin olive oil.

Cucumber and tomato salad.

Fresh fruit.

DINNER: DAY 6

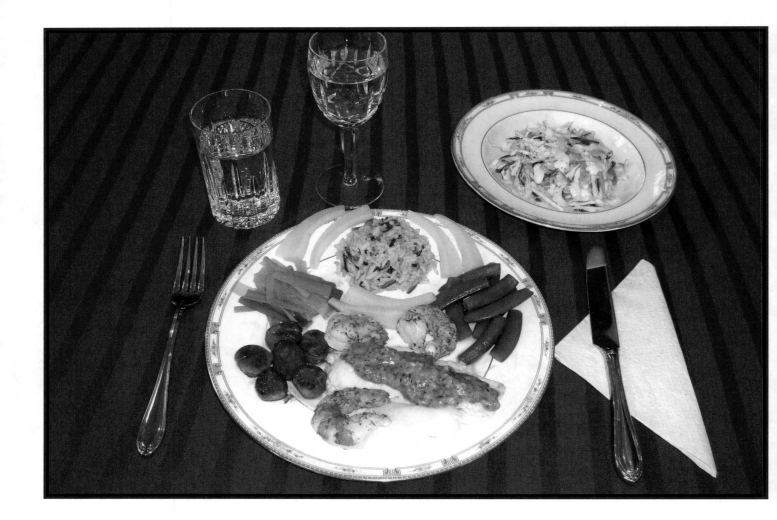

Any white ocean fish poached as in the day 2 salmon meal, with a spoon of seafood sauce (recipe shown on next page). Serve with shrimp cooked in a touch of dry white wine with lemon juice, cilantro, dill, fine herbs. To complete add some pan seared sea scallops cooked in olive oil after marinating in a combination of mushroom soya sauce, Maggi, and Worcestershire sauce.

Brown rice and wild rice cooked in low sodium chicken stock.

Steamed leeks, snow peas, green beans, and parsnips.

Cole slaw.

Fresh fruit.

DOUGIE'S HOMEMADE SEAFOOD SAUCE RECIPE

While this recipe has some drawbacks in terms of a healthy choice, you can make a large batch, and then freeze it in small bags to be used when necessary. A little bit will not harm you and it adds a lot of taste to the meal.

- 1 can low sodium cream of mushroom soup
- 1/4 cup of light mayonnaise
- 1/4 cup of capers
- 1 tablespoon of lemon juice
- 1 tablespoon of Dijon mustard
- 1 tablespoon of grated lemon peel
- 1/4 cup fine chop fresh mushrooms
- 1/4 cup Chardonnay wine or other dry white wine
- 3 tablespoons dried spinach
- 3 cloves fresh garlic fine chop
- 1 tablespoon Worcestershire sauce
- 1/4 teaspoon pepper
- 3-4 thin slices of gouda cheese
- 1/2 small onion or French shallots fine chop and cook in a little butter before adding to the sauce
- Add basil, cilantro, dill (go easy), and fine herbs to suit your taste
- Simmer for 20 minutes, stirring occasionally

DINNER: DAY 7

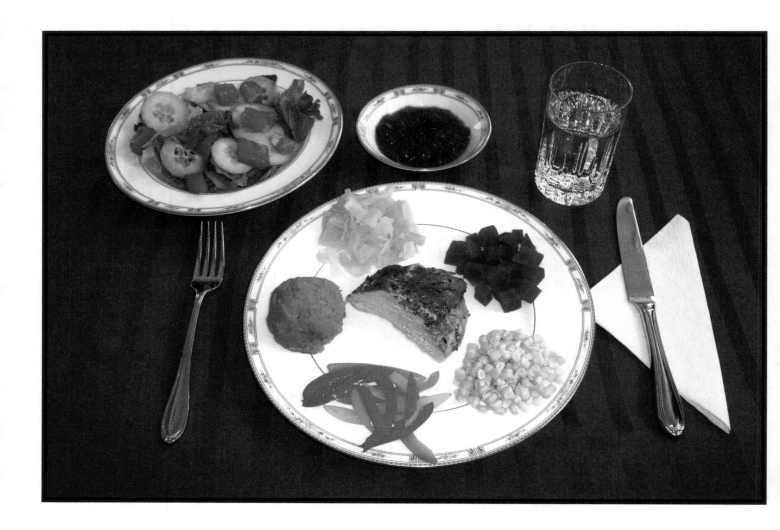

Roast turkey (20 minutes per pound).

One spoonful whole berry cranberry sauce.

Whipped sweet potato with a light sprinkle of salt and pepper.

Corn, cabbage, beets, and sweet peppers (red, orange, yellow).

Mixed green salad with oil and vinegar or small amount of low fat dressing.

Fresh fruit.

VARIATIONS AND MEAL NOTES

I am confident that you will thoroughly enjoy the foods being suggested in the menu. You can change up the vegetable combinations or salads to suit your own tastes. I recommend that you do not overdo the carrots, corn and peas because they are higher in sugar. A combination of your exercise program and these healthy food choices will ensure that you can reach your targeted proper weight. If you followed the menu selection for an entire week and did all your exercising properly, then allow yourself just one meal a week where you can treat yourself. These "rule breaker treats" might be a small portion of white bread, white potatoes, dessert, or cheese, but never over indulge and just choose one or two of the restricted items as a treat for your week of good habits. One glass of wine will not be overly harmful on this special day as you celebrate your accomplishments for the week.

You might also try making your own home made soups with any of the ingredients and spices shown above. Be creative and surprise yourself with some new cooking skills.

Once you have achieved your final weight goal, which will likely require several months, then you can take one dinner meal a week for a change in diet where you can experience some international cuisine. It would be a shame if you were not able to enjoy the unique foods created around the world and expand your culinary tastes. After your months of hard work and discipline, you have earned a much deserved respite. It is good to look forward to a small change in diet for one meal a week. This will improve your mental state, as you proved to yourself and others that you had what it takes to succeed. Just remember, do not overindulge and consume moderate amounts of food for this one meal. You do not want to revert back to your old habits and at your old weight.

Good luck!

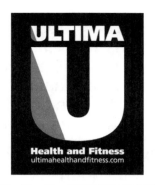

CHAPTER
7

VITAMIN AND MINERAL SUPPLEMENTS

The Council for Responsible Nutrition, which was founded in 1973, reported in 2002 that about one half of the U.S. population used dietary supplements. Sales of supplements have grown more than 5% per year over the past four years and now exceeds 9 billion dollars according to a 2010 4th edition report on National Supplements in the U.S. Clearly there is a growing trend in the regular use of supplements.

The growth in the supplement industry can be linked to people being more health conscious and wanting to ensure that they are ingesting sufficient vitamins and minerals to meet their daily needs. Our food supplies and the type of foods we choose to consume may not meet these nutritional needs. In addition, the prevalent use of nitrogen, phosphorous and potassium (NPK) fertilizers by our farmers means that the North American food supply and the food supply of many of the animals that we consume, have reduced value as a result of lower quality soils. Because of lower quality food sources that fail to provide the necessary nutritional base we require, there are likely benefits to topping up your daily vitamin and mineral requirements with supplements. While I personally believe that vitamin and mineral supplements have assisted me in my physical development, there are still many experts who maintain that our food sources can supply all of our bodies' nutritional needs. I am not convinced that our current food supply meets those needs due to the fairly extensive use of NPK's, pesticides, herbicides and food processing systems. If you want to be certain that you are consuming required levels of vitamins and minerals, then topping up your diet with supplements is a better option, in my view, than guessing as to whether or not you are getting all you need from food sources. Statistics from a 2008 report by the U.S. National Poison Control concluded that there were zero deaths from the consumption of vitamin and mineral supplements, so you should not be concerned about the toxicity of these supplements. That being said, it is still advisable to be reasonable in the amounts of supplements you consume based on your existing diet. Personally, I have been using a vitamin and mineral supplement program for over 18 years and have had no known side effects.

The next issue to be concerned about is obtaining quality supplement products and in amounts that meet your body's needs. When I first started using supplements, I would have a myriad of bottles that held each vitamin and mineral supplement separately. It was a time consuming, bulky, and annoying task to research and purchase so many different products. It is a much easier task to let scientific experts put together a combination of products that can be placed in daily packages. I like simplicity, consistency, and quality in my life, so I chose to use prepackaged daily AM and PM supplement packs over 18 years ago and got rid of the dozens of bottles of supplements. It was an easy decision but you need to ensure that your supplier is knowledgeable and is providing quality supplement products in proper dosages. Your supplement packages should also clarify if they are to be taken in the morning or evening to ensure their maximum effectiveness. After much research, I chose Dr. Michael Colgan as my supplier of vitamin packs. Dr. Colgan has exceptional international credentials in the fields of nutrition and physical training and has written over 15 books and numerous articles for leading nutritional publications. Throughout his illustrious 40 year career, he has also mentored and guided hundreds of professional and Olympic performers (including world champions) to help them significantly improve their performances. He offers wisdom, knowledge and experience to those of us who need guidance, and who are overwhelmed by the vast amounts of information directed at the consumer through advertising and marketing programs.

Lyle MacWilliams (MSc,FP) has written a book entitled "Nutrisearch – A Comparative Guide to Nutritional Supplements," which compared over 1500 manufacturers' products and ranked them in terms of quality. His book is now in its 4th edition, with the latest publication in 2009. He used NSF International to conduct the testing. NSF International started in 1974, and they are an independent, not-for-profit organization. They conducted tests of 1500 manufacturers' products in the NSF laboratories to ensure that the actual contents of the product match those on the labeling. NSF also confirmed that all ingredients were disclosed, and that there were no contaminants in the products. Third party research – that is, research not conducted by the manufacturers themselves – is important, as the results should be as unbiased as possible. Colgan Institute Mens or Womens Paks, and Sports Pak (AM/PM vitamin packs) are ranked among the top six suppliers offering combination supplement packs, so I believe I made the right choice over 18 years ago.

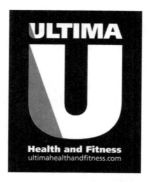

CHAPTER
8

PAIN MANAGEMENT AND SLEEP MANAGEMENT

Early in my initial training, I began to make remarkable progress on one particular exercise - a cable pull down behind the neck to the shoulders. I experienced some elbow pain at first, but I grinned and bared it and eventually I was able to pull down the entire stack of weights. I felt really good about myself and even the "big boys" in the gym were impressed. Week after week, my elbow joints became increasingly painful, but I persisted in pulling the whole stack just to prove to myself and others that I was getting stronger. Eventually the pain was so intense that I would lay in bed at night with both elbows throbbing. I finally relented and went for physiotherapy. During my physiotherapy, I discovered that I had damaged the tendons on both of my arms on the inside and outside elbow joints. I had medial and lateral epicondylitis in both arms. This is more commonly known as tennis elbow and golfer's elbow. The solution was several months of therapy three times a week and no upper body training. Ultimately, the therapy was not successful and the doctor recommended cortisone shots as the last option to solve the problem. I ended up getting a total of six cortisone shots – three for each elbow joint. They were very painful but after a few weeks the elbow joints felt well and I started training my upper body again.

Once I began retraining, I committed myself to a practice that I still follow to this day and it is now my advice to you. If you have an injury or if an exercise results in too much pain – just stop! Get medical help from your physician, physiotherapist, chiropractor, or acupuncturist, and let your body heal. I cannot tell you how many people I have seen over the years who work through the pain and learn to regret their decision years later when there is either no solution for their injury, or major surgery is required.

You can continue to do other exercise routines for the same body part that does not lead to pain. Later in this book you will see a multitude of exercises that can be performed for each body part. Then, once you are able to return to the exercise that caused your injury, work your way back slowly to ensure you do not repeat the same problem. By using these principles, I have avoided any serious injury for over 17 years without having to compromise the quality of my fitness routines. You do not want to enter old age with a body that is wracked with pain due to injuries that were not managed properly. You may want to consider using a quality Glucosamine Sulphate supplement to assist you in times of joint pain. This product is actually already included in my daily vitamin packs, which I have been using for many years, and despite a pretty rigorous training routine, I do not have any joint pain after 17 years of pretty intense training.

THE IMPORTANCE OF SLEEP

You spend approximately one third of your life in bed. Because so much time is spent in bed sleeping, you should make sure that you have a top quality mattress that supports proper posture and pillows that help provide you with a good nights rest. If you are tired because of a poor mattress or uncomfortable pillows, your day-to-day life and your exercise routines will suffer greatly. You will not have the energy you need to perform to the best of your abilities, whether it is at work or at the gym. While I acknowledge that the initial cost of a new mattress is high, consider it to be a long-term investment for your own well being, and make it a priority issue. You should also be getting at least 7 to 8 hours of sleep each night to ensure maximum performance during your busy day schedule.

For those of you who have difficulty sleeping, I have personally found success with Douglas Laboratories low dosages of melatonin. However, it is important to discuss any and all sleep assistance options with a medical professional to weigh the benefits and risks associated with such medications.

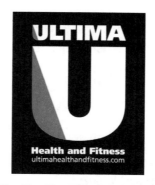

CHAPTER
9

PERFORMANCE ENHANCING DRUGS

Let me make my position crystal clear about the use of performance enhancing drugs and other illegal performance enhancing techniques such as blood doping: I am totally against their use in any dosage, for any amount of time, excluding legal prescriptions, for medical purposes only. I would like to see much more stringent rules to control their use, both inside and outside the sports arena.

My male sports heroes are people like Wayne Gretzky, Michael Jordan, Bruce Lee, Roberto Clemente, Henry Aaron, and Babe Ruth. They took their natural talent and spent years honing their skills to become some of the greatest athletes the world has ever seen. How about Sugar Ray Robinson, arguably the best boxer of all time. His amateur record was 85 and 0 and in the first eleven years of his professional career, he posted a 128 - 1- and 2 record. Then there was Paavo Nurmi who set 25 world records, and held 9 gold medals and 3 silver medals in three Olympics in the 1920s and 1930s. The great Canadian Louis Cyr is arguably the strongest man who ever lived. He lifted over 4000 lbs on a back lift and did a one handed dumbbell dead lift with 525 lbs in the late 1800s. None of these great athletes had to use the crutch of performance enhancing drugs to establish their historical credentials. We need more honest and true champions like these to revere.

The underlying principle that seems to be at the forefront of sports today is "winning is everything" and athletes will "do whatever it takes" to gain fame and fortune and to achieve an unfair advantage over their adversaries. So many top athletes in both the Olympics and professional sports have been caught using performance enhancing drugs. Most often, their first response is that they did not cheat. Great lesson they are teaching our youth – first lie and deny, then relent and repent. Hollow words indeed. The corporate world of sports was, for many years, more focused on filling the seats rather than solving a drug problem involving their players that they almost certainly knew existed. The situation has improved, but not to the extent that it should. There are still too many cheats. Too often, it is not the best athlete who comes out on top – it is the athlete with the best chemist. It is a very disturbing trend that has only become worse in terms of the number of athletes around the world who are following this path. This has to be devastating to the honest athlete who likely spends in excess of 10 or 15 years trying to be the best without chemical assistance.

That trend translates into use of performance enhancing drugs outside the sports field and into the daily lives of our young people who look up to their heroes for direction and inspiration. Please refer to the U.S. Department of Justice Drug Enforcement Administration publication on "Steroid Abuse in Today's Society" (published March, 2004). That publication underlies how widespread the steroid problem has become. What is most disturbing is that products like steroids, human growth hormone and ephedrine are sold openly on the Internet on North American websites. Since these products are all controlled substances, they can only be legally obtained by prescription and should technically not be available to the general public. Despite the difficulties of tracking down and punishing online sellers (especially when sellers cross boundaries, making it difficult to know which country is responsible for punishment), I think it is necessary to crack down on illegal selling of performance enhancing drugs. If the public sees little or no consequences to individuals dealing or consuming illegal substances, then the problem is unlikely to improve. There needs to be some serious financial and jailing consequences to illegal drug marketing in order to see a change for the better. Extensive testing in professional sports is another necessity in order to stop the abuse of performance enhancing drugs. Professional sports make up a multi billion dollar industry that, in many cases, pays astronomical wages to its players. To say that it will be too expensive to carry out tests on a much more rigorous scale seems like a poorly justifiable excuse. Players unions also need to get onside with the concept of increased drug testing to improve the integrity of professional sports.

The man who brought steroids to North America in 1958 was Dr. John Zeigler. He set off a litany of steroid usage that resulted in the premature deaths of hundreds of athletes, mostly due to heart failure. Zeigler himself died of heart failure at the relatively young age of 63 and had turned against the use of steroids once he saw the damages caused by its use. Bodybuilder Mike Mentzer and wrestling star "Ravishing Rick Rude" never made it to the age of 50. Their hearts gave out due to steroid use. If you want to learn more about the terrible consequences of steroid use, consult the website *www. athletesagainststeroids.org*. To me the analogy is like the anorexic who looks in the mirror and says "I'm way too big," while the steroid user looks in the mirror and says "I'm not big enough". Both represent a view which is far too extreme and dangerous to their health.

Steroids reduce your high-density lipoprotein (known as HDL or the "good cholesterol") and increase your low-density lipoprotein (known as LDL or the "bad cholesterol"), which can cause major heart problems. Steroids are proven to enlarge the prostrate and damage your liver. So why would anyone want to use a substance that has proven serious side effects? The shortsighted goals of fame and fortune often blind individuals to what is best for them in the long term.

The latest "fad" in performance enhancing drugs is Human Growth Hormone (HGH), which has been around since the 1980s. Once again, it is a controlled substance that should only be available by legal prescription. The reality is that this drug is being used extensively in the sports arena, as acknowledged by the U.S. Department of Justice Drug Enforcement Administration on their website. You can review their website to learn about several adverse side effects.

Another type of drug problem involves blood doping using Erythropoietin (EPO) and has occurred a great deal in the cycling world. The number of charges for using this illegal technique has grown over the years as drug testing increasingly looked for the use of EPO. In 1998 almost 50% of the riders in the Tour De France pulled out of the race after an EPO drug scandal was exposed at the highest level. There have been a number of deaths of elite cyclists in their 20s and 30s that are linked to EPO use. I personally have completely lost interest in following cycling as a result of these scandals.

SUCCESS WITHOUT PERFORMANCE ENHANCING DRUGS

Chest exercises are my weakest routine and I always dreamed of performing a flat bench press with 225 lbs. I spent years trying to reach this goal. It never happened, and my personal best was performing a flat bench of 205 lbs, which I reached in my mid-50s. However, I was able to perform many other weight training and cardio routines that most people my size, regardless of their age, would struggle to complete. I could look into the mirror every morning and know that I had given my best. I never sacrificed my moral integrity for a result that could have been achieved by using performance enhancing drugs. A former bodybuilder who was a regular member at the gym I attended had watched for years how hard I trained, and when he saw the heavy weights I was able to lift, he said, "Dougie, if you ever went on juice, you would be scary". True story – I would have been scary! But by training hard and avoiding the pitfalls of drug use, I was able to put my HDL cholesterol levels in the top 5 of 2000 patients seen by my personal physician - and I was able to do this at the age of 58! Now that's making real progress in the betterment of your long-term health. So if you want good long term health and well being, stay away from performance enhancing drugs.

For anyone who wants to change their direction in life, never underestimate the power of the human spirit to overcome what appear to be overwhelming odds. I can point to two examples of historical figures who made their mark with their incredible achievements despite the seemingly impossible odds they were forced to overcome. The first is the famous French painter Pierre Auguste Renoir, who is one of my favourite artists. He was so badly crippled with arthritis that his hands were grossly deformed, he was wheel-chair bound, and he could barely hold a paint brush. Yet he persevered and despite his limitations, he continued to create masterpieces. The second example is my motor racing hero Tazio Nuvolari who was the lead driver for two of the greatest race car builders in history – Enzo Ferrari and Dr. Ferdinand Porsche. In one of Nuvolari's most famous European Grand Prix races, he had to compete against 7 other leading competitors who had 50% more horsepower and a better designed chassis. That is a huge advantage and in today's racing world it would be practically impossible to qualify for the race. Yet Nuvolari defeated them all by outdriving them. Take stock from these examples. You can, and will, achieve much more than you can ever imagined with effort and perseverance.

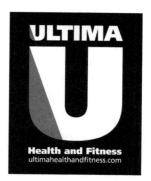

CHAPTER
10

TRAINING BASICS, SCHEDULES AND ROUTINE OPTIONS

TRAINING ROUTINES

I firmly believe that any healthy training program must include stretching, abdominals, and cardio as basics. Weight training alone should not dominate your program. As you age, you will lose your flexibility and endurance, especially if you avoid stretches and cardio work. Cardio is necessary to strengthen your heart, burn off fat, and increase lung capacity amongst many other benefits. Your best long-term health routine should consistently include all these basics each time you exercise. The best time to train is in the morning, or early afternoon if possible. Training late at night can play havoc on your sleep pattern, so if you only are able to train in the evenings, make it sooner rather than later in the evening.

After years of experimenting with different combinations, I have created a weight training routine that I personally found to be the most effective. Details of the routine are found under the heading "Suggested Weight Training Schedule". Since we are all made differently, you will have to adjust your own weight training routine to maximize your performance and make the most of your time at the gym. Keep trying different combinations to discover which one provides you with the best results. It may take you several months to finally find the right combination. Keep notes on your progress to help you find that perfect balance of routines for maximum performance. Initially I tried to work out 5 days a week in a row for two hours a day, but I found it was too exhausting. I fell into overtraining and was losing weight on a small frame. Don't fall into this trap. Part of being healthy is knowing when not to overdo it at the gym.

BASIC TRAINING SCHEDULE

I begin every workout with stretches, followed by shoulder warm up exercises and abdominal exercises. I follow these warm-ups and abdominals with my regular weight training and finish with at least 20 minutes of hard cardio. I feel that this workout regime provides me with the best results. I tried doing cardio earlier in my routine, but found that I was not able to perform my weight training at the intensity I desired. Doing abdominals at the end of the program was a write off because I could simply not perform the routines properly, as my energy level for that muscle group had been expended during weight training. In order to achieve the results I wanted, the abs had to be done early on in the program.

SUGGESTED WEIGHT TRAINING SCHEDULE

- Day 1: Chest only
- Day 2: Biceps and Triceps
- Day 3: Rest or cardio/abs
- Day 4: Back and Shoulders
- Day 5: Legs
- Day 6: Rest
- Day 7: Rest

I suggest a minimum of two days a week to rest so that you do not strain or exhaust your body. When you choose to take these two days is up to you. I recommend experimenting to see where the rests in your schedule provide the best results when you return to the gym.

WATER HYDRATION

You must sip water before stretching, after stretching, between all abdominal routines, between each set of weight training routines, and during cardio exercises. It is extremely important to keep your muscles hydrated in order to achieve maximum performance. I consumed at least one and a half to two liters of water during my workout. Remember to use clean water, as outlined in Chapter 5.

HOW MUCH TIME EXERCISING

The length of time you will spend in the gym on the days you train will depend on your endurance level. After a year of training, I had built up my endurance and would spend two hours training on each workout day. I was able to do this without feeling exhausted or worn out, despite a fairly rigorous exercise program. Once again, everyone is different and you need to experiment to see how far you can push the envelope. You may find that one hour is all you can take without being run down, and that's fine. Just be sure that you do the mandatory routines outlined above (stretching, abdominals and cardio), and spend less time on weight training.

CONTROL YOUR TRAINING ENVIRONMENT

All weight training routines must use smooth, controlled body movements, focusing on the body part being exercised. Bouncing weights off of your body, or twisting your body in strange contortions just to complete a routine is not effective and can lead to serious injury. When I am in the process of weight training, I try to go from the start position to the end position quickly but with control, and then slow it down on the return to the start position. If you are lifting very heavy weights, you should always have another gym member spot you to make sure that you are capable of completing your routine. I have seen a number of people get injured because they failed to have a spotter in place when they were unable to complete a lift. Also, be careful who you use as a spotter - make sure that they have experience because the use of an inexperienced spotter can result in an injury.

RESTING

Stretching exercises should be done without resting, moving from one exercise to the next until all routines are done. You should take a one-minute rest between abdominal exercise routines. Rest at least two to three minutes between chest exercises to allow your body to recover. For the bicep-triceps combination, you can do a bicep routine followed immediately by a triceps routine, and then take a two-minute rest between the next two bicep-triceps combination. You are able to do these combination routines because you are involving two different muscle groups: one pulling (biceps) and one pushing (triceps). The same applies to the back-shoulders combination – do one then the other immediately. Again the same concept applies – back is a pulling exercise and shoulders are a pushing exercise. Rest two to three minutes between each combination set of back and shoulders because this is a larger muscle group and needs more time to recover. For leg routines, you should rest between two and three minutes between sets to fully recover. You might like to try combination leg extensions (works the quad muscles on the front of the leg) and then immediately hamstrings (works muscles on the backs of the legs). You will still likely need a rest between sets if you are doing heavier weights. These can sap your energy level if done with intensity.

PYRAMID TRAINING

I have used pyramid training on most training days, which involves doing three or four sets of each weight training routine as follows:

- Set 1: 10 repetitions

- Set 2: 6 to 8 repetitions with heavier weights
- Set 3: 2 to 4 repetitions with close to your maximum capabilities
- Set 4: 1 repetition of your maximum capability

Pyramid training will provide you with additional strength as you begin to progress with heavier weights.

HEAVY NEGATIVES

Heavy negatives will give you much more power. This procedure involves doing weight training with weights heavier than you can normally lift. One or two spotters must be used to lift the initial weight (which is normally beyond your capabilities) to place the weight on your body while you hold your start position. Once the weight is in place, you will slowly return to the finish position, counting slowly backwards from 5. You must be in total body control while returning to the finish position. The spotters will then return the weights to the start position with no help from yourself. Only go slightly above your normal weight capabilities and do not go beyond your limitations to the point of injuring yourself. When performing heavy negatives, you must remember that you will only be able to do a few repetitions. Using a Smith machine with stop positions can take the risk out of heavy negatives for chest and shoulder routines. Make certain that you initially add only 10% more weight over your maximum lift, and then increase that up to 20% over time. This is a routine where you must know and trust your spotters, or serious injury can result. I would not recommend using heavy negatives for a long period. Your body will need a rest after a few weeks of this intensity, and you can either take a break from heavy negatives by performing your regular weight training, or by modifying your weight training by using lighter weights. Even while on a break from heavy negatives, be sure to continue with stretches, abdominals and cardio.

DROP SETS

Drop sets will give you more endurance. This procedure involves doing a routine as follows with no rest between sets:

Set 1: 10 repetitions with about 80% of your maximum weight capability

Set 2: 10 repetitions with about 60% of your maximum weight capability

Set 3: 10 repetitions, or to failure, with about 50% of your maximum weight capability

Similar to heavy negatives, I would not recommend drop sets for the long term. Also, I would use drop sets for one or two routines per body part on any training day to avoid overtraining.

CIRCUIT TRAINING

Circuit training involves the training of all your muscle groups by constantly moving from one body part routine to another using reduced weights. In performing circuit training, you take a very short rest between each exercise routine. Here are the steps for circuit training:

1. **Choose one exercise routine per chapter from chapters 15 to 18**

2. **Using reduced weights, do one routine for each body part, moving quickly from one body part to another until all body parts have been exercised**

3. **Take a break for 2 or 3 minutes**

4. **Begin again at step 1, selecting new routines for each body part from the chapters listed.**

Circuit training can be used by beginners (using very little weights, so as not to overload the body), as well as experienced trainers who have taken time off from the gym and want to warm up all their muscle groups. For experienced trainers, circuit training gives the body time to readjust to heavier stresses on the body once more serious training takes place in a week or so. Circuit training may be a solution for those who have extreme time constraints in the gym and still want to work on all their body parts. However, it does not have the full benefits of much more strenuous routines, and I rarely use circuit training myself.

I recommend, of course, that you always continue with the same core exercises mentioned earlier – stretches and abdominals before the circuit raining, followed by cardio.

PROTEIN INTAKE

For many years, I ensured that I had a protein shake after every training routine. I also made sure that I was using a top quality iso whey protein in my shakes. I have to say, in retrospect, they did nothing for me. I never gained a single pound and I tended to feel bloated after consuming the shake. I stopped having protein shakes altogether and never found an ounce of difference in either my performance or my weight fluctuation. I know there are many experts and athletes who swear by protein supplements and shakes, but I have yet to personally see the benefits these products offer. Based on the careful planning of my diet, I can only assume that my meals include sufficient protein to handle my body's needs. I suggest you try a program with a whey protein supplement followed by a program without the supplement and after training for a few months using each method, see if you are receiving any benefit from the added protein.

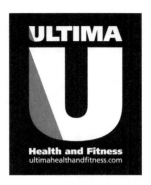

CHAPTER
11

FREE WEIGHTS VERSUS MACHINES

There is certainly no question that free weights - defined as weights not connected to a machine, such as dumbbells and barbells - help to develop the stabilizer muscles that are constantly called upon when you are in the sports arena. As such, if you are involved with competitive sports then free weights are very important in the physical development of your smaller stabilizer muscles, as well as the development of larger muscle mass. While free weights have obvious benefits, it is important to also recognize the possibility of injury using free weights and knowing how to avoid such injuries. I have seen many people get serious injuries while training with free weights and most of these people had years of experience and training. You want to ensure that you do proper stretching and other warm-up exercises that help to prevent injuries. Later chapters deal with preventative measures to avoid injury, as well as instructions to perform a number of safe and effective free weight exercise routines.

As you age, you want a more stable environment to carry out your exercises and I am a supporter of some machines that are used for weight training to provide for that stable environment. I acknowledge that these machines are not as effective as free weights to develop your body for competitive sports since they typically do not work the stabilizer muscles. The machines I suggest are outlined in later chapters for each body part. After 18 years of observation, I have yet to see anyone injured in the gym while exercising on the machines that I recommend.

Please note that I am not in favor of doing any abdominal exercise that requires a machine. I consider most abdominal machines to be marketing gimmicks that do not work. If you use the abdominal exercises recommended in this book as opposed to commercially available machines, I am confident that you will achieve much better results.

FITNESS MODELS

SUSAN ARRUDA BIO

IBRAHIM KAMAL BIO

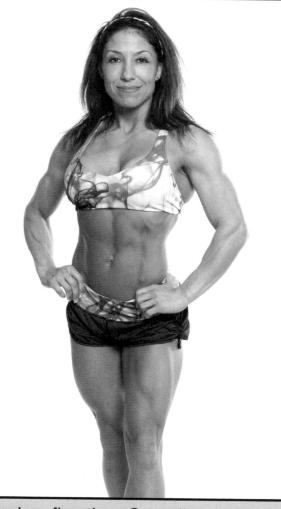

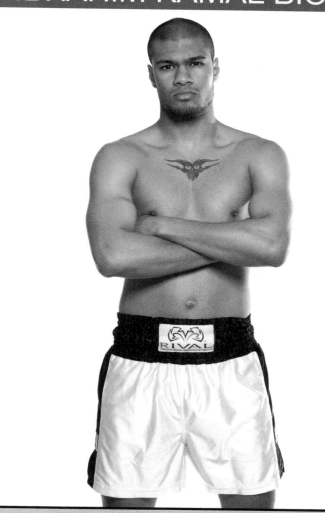

Susan is a five time Canadian National Figure Champion. She is the 2009 WBFF World Championships double title first place winner, and also the first place Figure Category FAME World and Nationals Championships winner for three consecutive years from 2006 onward. Susan holds PRO cards in both federations. More remarkable, Susan is also a 42 year old mother of two who has been training naturally for over 30 years. You can visit Susan's website at www.seriouscurvestraining. com to learn more about Susan and her many accomplishments and the experience that she brings to the fitness world.

Ibrahim is the eight time Canadian National Amateur Boxing Champion. He took up boxing at a young age to stop being bullied. He went on to spend his entire amateur career at Cabbagetown Boxing Club in Toronto. Ibrahim has now turned professional and as an amateur has beaten every one of the current top ranked professional Canadian Lightweight boxers. He plans to take the Canadian Professional Lightweight Boxing Title in the near future.

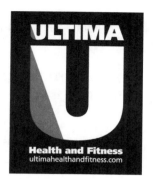

CHAPTER
12
STRETCHES

Stretching has been proven to reduce injuries and improve flexibility, so it is a key exercise to perform before you begin training or competing in any sport. It is also important to ensure that you are stretching all of the appropriate parts of your body that will be called on once you begin to stress the body. You can perform one stretch after another with no rest between stretches to avoid taking too much time to perform all the necessary stretches. That being said, you need to remember some basic strategies when performing your stretches.

1. You should be relaxed and stretch to a point where there is tension, but not discomfort. When you first begin, your range of motion may be limited and that is to be expected. As time progresses, you can gently increase the range of your stretch. Do not be intimidated by some of the stretches shown in the photos of this chapter – with time and effort, you will be able to duplicate (or come close to duplicating) the range of motion shown. Remember that the person in the photo has spent years obtaining her flexibility.

2. Breathe normally during the stretch.

3. The stretch should last at least 30 seconds.

4. Move from one stretch to the other with only a few seconds rest between each stretch. You do not want to take up too much of your gym time stretching at the

expense of abdominal and weight training, which require resting between sets. Make the most of your time in the gym.

5. Use a mat designed for floor stretches. Gym floors are generally pretty firm and make for an uncomfortable environment to perform your stretches.

Thirty years ago, a physiotherapist taught me the first three stretches shown below. I had spent four years getting treatments for a lower back rotational injury I incurred from playing football. I tried several different therapists and chiropractors to attempt to solve the problem over the course of four years and none of the treatments helped. During that time, I was in a lot of discomfort and had limited motion. Once I was taught these three lower back stretches, and worked on them daily, it only took about three months to completely eradicate the lower back problem. These three stretches in particular are excellent for stretching lower back muscles.

LOWER BACK STRETCH

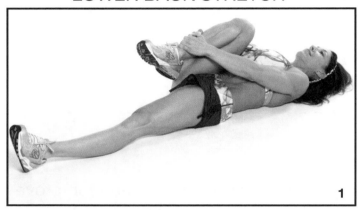

1. PULL FIRMLY AT YOUR ANKLE, AND CONCENTRATE ON PUSHING DOWN THE SMALL OF YOUR BACK INTO THE FLOOR

LOWER BACK STRETCH

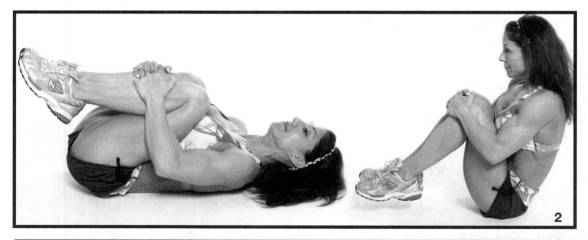

2. START POSITION - PULL YOUR KNEES TIGHTLY TO YOUR CHEST
FINISH POSITION - ROLL FRONTWARDS TO REST YOUR FEET ON THE FLOOR TOGETHER

LOWER BACK STRETCH

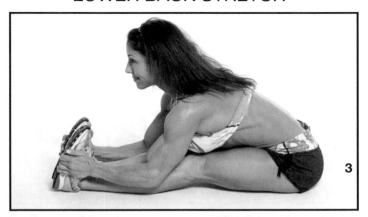

3. REACH AS FAR TO YOUR TOES AS POSSIBLE OR BEYOND IF YOU ARE CAPABLE WITH BOTH HANDS

YOGA STRETCH

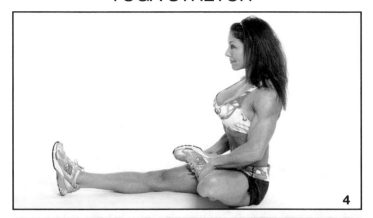

4. KEEPING ONE LEG STRAIGHT, PULL THE OTHER OVER GENTLY TWISTING THE ANKLE UPWARD

REACH FOR THE SKY

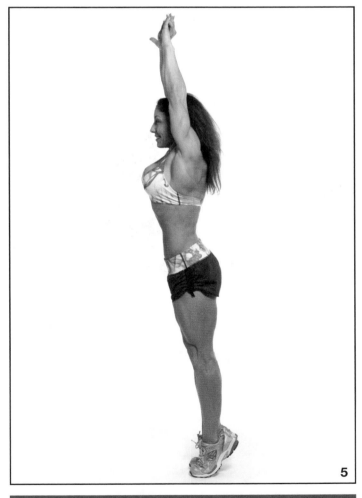

5. LOCK YOUR THUMBS TOGETHER AND REACH AS HIGH AS YOU POSSIBLY CAN REACH

BACKWARD LEAN

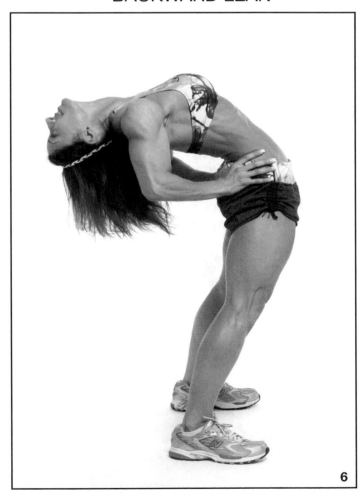

6. YOU MAY BE MORE COMFORTABLE USING A WALL AS A REFERENCE POINT BEHIND YOU FOR SAFETY

ABDUCTOR STRETCH

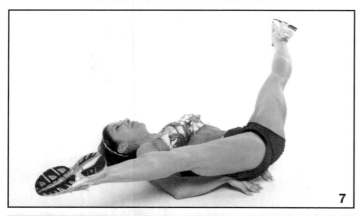

7. NOTE POSITION OF HANDS SUPPORTING LOWER BODY

HAMSTRING STRETCH

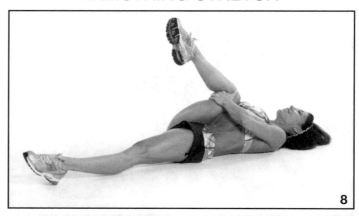

8. PULL VERY FIRMLY BENEATH THE KNEE TO YOUR CHEST

BODY TWIST

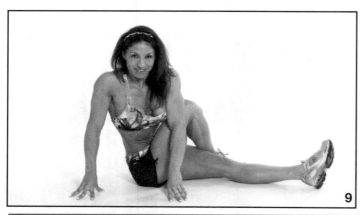

9. NOTE POSITION OF BOTH HANDS AND LEGS - SWITCH SIDES AFTER 30 SECONDS

MACKENZIE STRETCH

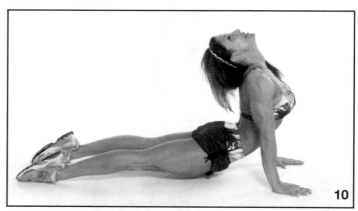

10. DO NOT LET YOUR HIPS TOUCH THE FLOOR TO GET A MAXIMUM STRETCH

SIDE STRETCH

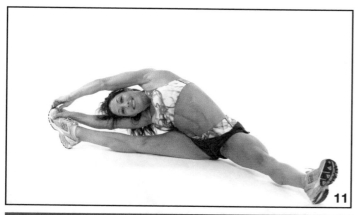

11. REACH WITH BOTH HANDS AS FAR AS POSSIBLE TO ONE SIDE - SWITCH SIDES AFTER 30 SECONDS

HIP ROTATION

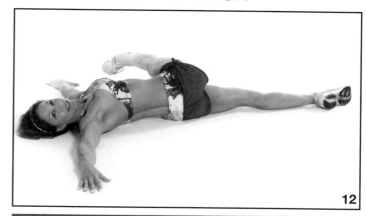

12. ARMS IN CROSS POSITION ON FLOOR, ONE LEG STRAIGHT, THE OTHER ROTATED TO OPPOSITE SIDE - SWITCH SIDES AFTER 30 SECONDS

BALLET STRETCH

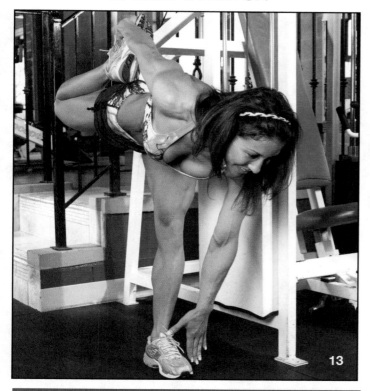

13. YOU CAN DO THIS SUPPORTED BY HOLDING ON TO A PIECE OF EQUIPMENT, OR UNSUPPORTED SEEN HERE

ANKLE, HAMSTRING, SHOULDER STRETCH

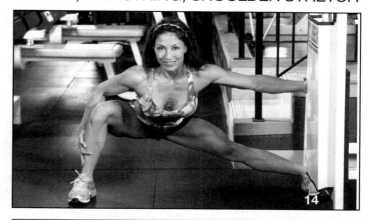

14. PLACE FOOT AGAINST BOTTOM OF EQUIPMENT FOR SUPPORT OF ANKLE BEING STRETCHED - SWITCH SIDES AFTER 30 SECONDS

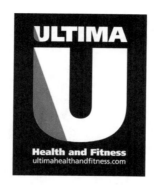

CHAPTER
13
SHOULDER WARM-UPS

The ball and socket joints - being the shoulders and hips - are the most flexible joints in the body. These joints allow your arms and legs to move freely. But the shoulder has the disadvantage of having a much smaller socket and stabilizer muscles than the hips to handle heavy stress. I can tell you of dozens of stories of experienced weight trainers who literally ruined their training careers because of shoulder injuries that could have likely been prevented with proper shoulder warm ups. Many of these injuries required surgery and even after the surgery many of the injured individuals I knew were limited in what they could perform. You can limit your exposure to such injuries by performing shoulder warm ups on every training day. These warm ups do not require a lot of time each time you do them, but they will be highly beneficial in the future of your training. I have not had a single problem with my shoulders despite heavy lifting on a regular basis.

When performing cable exercises, start with relatively light weights to begin and then slowly add more weight as weeks and months go by to the point where there is reasonable stress on the muscles. Please do not use heavy weights - this is a warm up exercise and stabilizer building routine, not heavy duty weight training.

You can do the exercises as shown in the following photos with no rest between each routine, thereby giving you more time for more strenuous exercises.

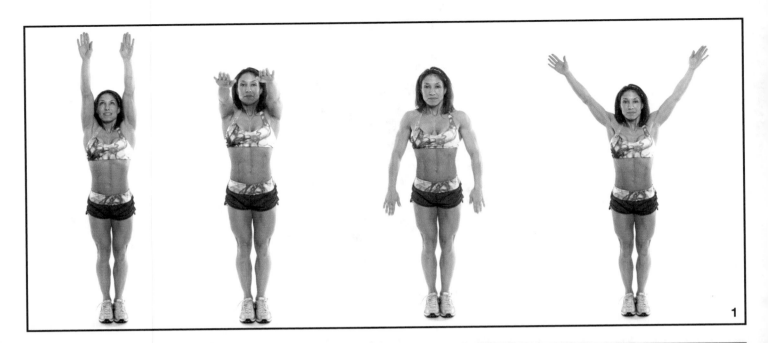

1. THIS MOVEMEMENT IS VERY SIMILAR TO DOING A BREASTSTROKE IN SWIMMING. DO A FULL SWING OF YOUR ARMS IN FRONT AND THEN BEHIND YOUR BACK . THEN AFTER 10 REPS, REVERSE THE MOTION SO THAT IT IS SIMILAR TO A DOUBLE ARM BACKSTROKE

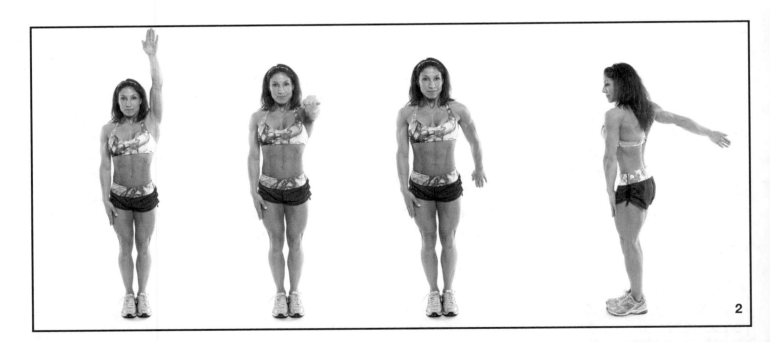

2. THIS MOVEMENT IS A SINGLE ARM WINDMILL MOVING YOUR ONE ARM IN A CIRCULAR MOTION

START POSITION   FINISH POSITION

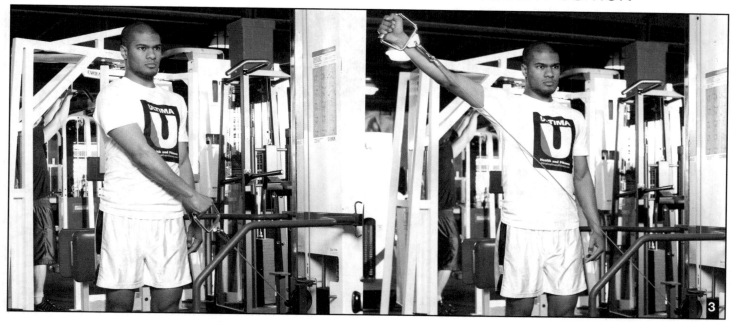

3. OUTWARD ROTATION, BOTTOM TO TOP - DO NOT BEND YOUR ARM DURING THIS MOVEMENT

START POSITION   FINISH POSITION

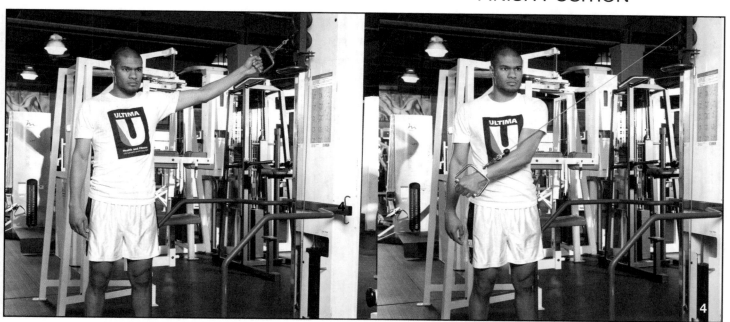

4. INWARD ROTATION, TOP TO BOTTOM - DO NOT BEND YOUR ARM DURING THIS MOVEMENT

START POSITION   FINISH POSITION

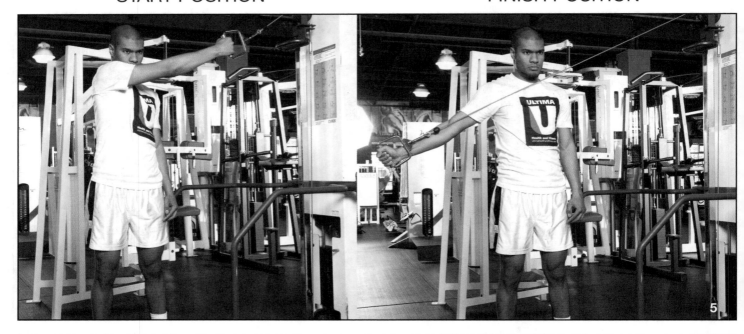

5. OUTWARD ROTATION, TOP TO BOTTOM - DO NOT BEND YOUR ARM DURING THIS MOVEMENT

START POSITION   FINISH POSITION

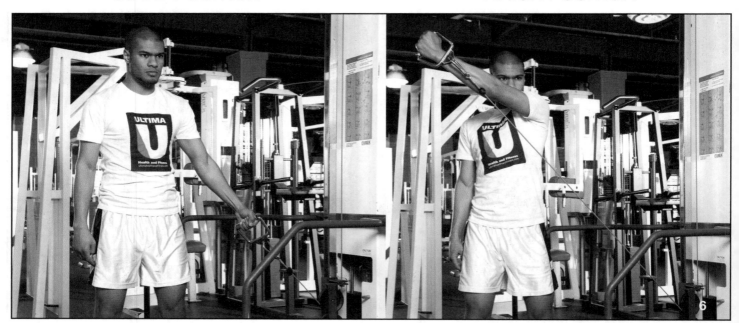

4. INWARD ROTATION, BOTTOM TO TOP - DO NOT BEND YOUR ARM DURING THIS MOVEMENT

START POSITION   FINISH POSITION

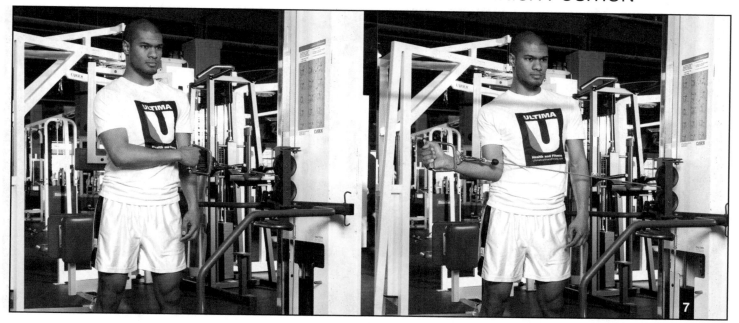

7. HORIZONTAL EXTERNAL ROTATION - NOTE THE POSITION OF THE ELBOW KEPT CLOSE TO YOUR BODY

START POSITION   FINISH POSITION

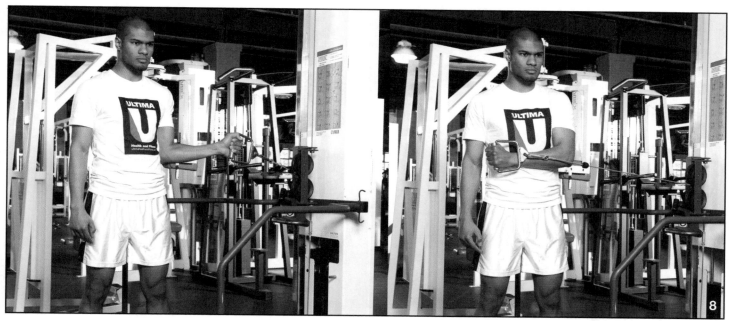

8. HORIZONTAL INTERNAL ROTATION - NOTE THE POSITION OF THE ELBOW KEPT CLOSE TO YOUR BODY

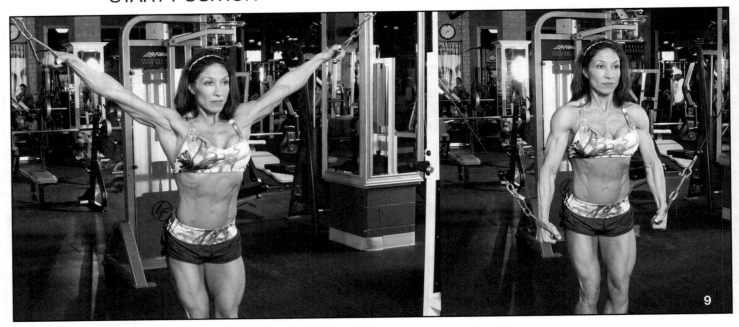

9. LATERAL CABLE PULL-DOWNS

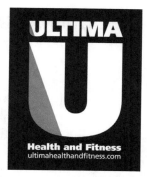

CHAPTER
14

ABDOMINAL AND LOWER BACK EXERCISES

Your abdominals and lower back are the very core of your body and are generally overlooked in exercise routines, or are not trained properly by most people. Your core supports your entire upper body and should be as strong as possible, especially if you are involved with competitive sports. A strong core will also help you in the development of your legs as you call on your core to support heavier weights.

The abdominal exercises shown in this book are proven to work, and I am living proof of that fact. The gym in which I trained for over 15 years had over 2000 members and even in my 60's I was a top performer when it came to abdominal routines, when compared to members in their 20s or 30s. If you follow this program, I am certain you will have one of the strongest abs in your gym.

I have divided the abdominal exercises into three groups that represent a building process. Once you are able to easily accomplish one phase of the building process, then move on to the next phase. To ensure proper form for beginner and intermediate ab routines and lower back exercises, follow the instructional photos featured in this chapter. For advanced ab routines, use the photos as a guide and be sure to consult the more detailed instructions with each photo.

BEGINNER ABDOMINAL ROUTINES

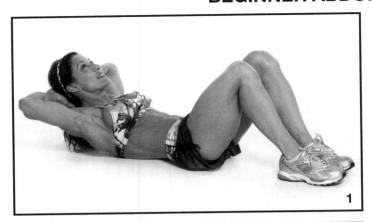

1. FLOOR CRUNCH WITH BOTH FEET FLAT ON THE FLOOR

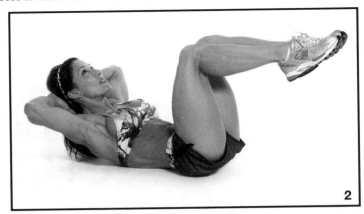

2. FLOOR CRUNCH WITH BOTH LEGS RAISED AT 90 DEGREE ANGLE

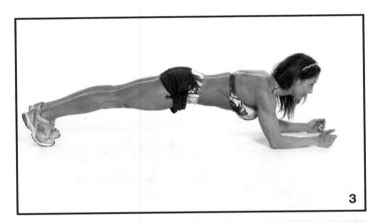

3. PLANK AB BASIC

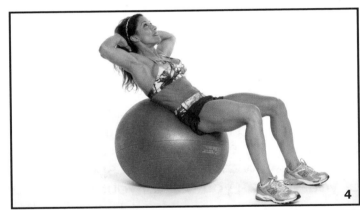

4. SWISS BALL CRUNCH

INTERMEDIATE ABDOMINAL ROUTINES

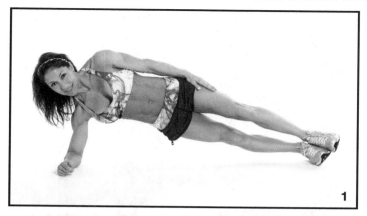

1. SIDE PLANK ABS

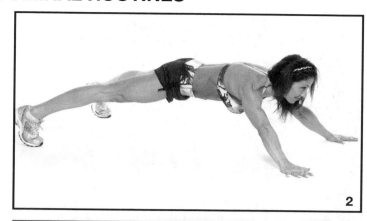

2. WIDE STANCE PLANK ABS

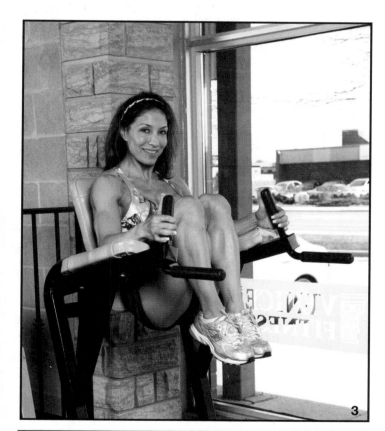

3. CAPTAINS CHAIR KNEE TO CHEST

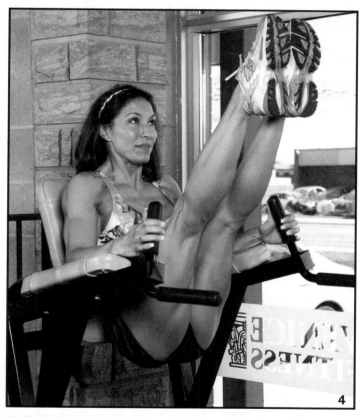

4. CAPTAINS CHAIR STRAIGHT LEG RAISE

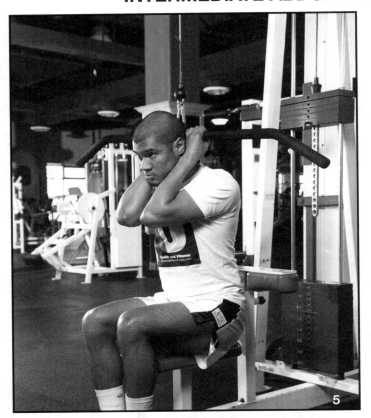

5. REVERSE CABLE CRUNCH WITH MEDIUM WEIGHTS - START POSITION

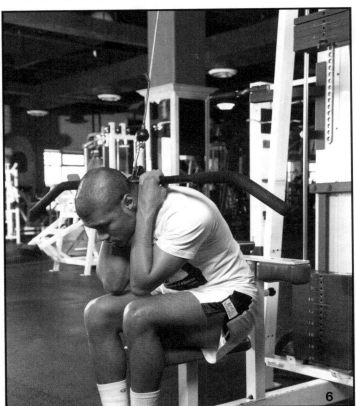

6. REVERSE CABLE CRUNCH WITH MEDIUM WEIGHTS - FINISH POSITION

ADVANCED ABDOMINAL ROUTINES

The "Loonie" (Centre Abs)

The "loonie" crunch (named after the Canadian one dollar coin) was an exercise I developed through years of experience after trying dozens of different abdominal routines. This one is unique, and it really knits your core together. If you do this exercise properly, you should feel immediate benefits to the centre of your abs. To perform the "loonie" crunch, lay flat on your back and place a loonie (or other coin) between your knees and put your lower legs at a right angle with your thighs in a vertical position. Touch your fingertips to the temples of your head and keep your elbows in tight; point your elbows toward your thighs. You need to make a *slow and concentrated movement* toward your thighs. About three inches from the upper thigh, exhale as much as possible and *squeeze the last three inches* to touch your upper thighs with the tips of your elbows. Throughout the routine be sure to: keep your elbows in tight, *use a controlled rhythmic movement*, exhale hard the last three inches just before you are actually touching the upper thighs with both elbow tips, do not move your thighs from the vertical position, and keep your knees tightly together. Drop the loonie and you are out of the game!

Hanging Leg Raises (Lower Abs)

To perform hanging leg raises, you must inhale before the raise up, and exhale on the movement back down to the start position. You should *not* swing your body during this routine. Your arms and shoulders must remain stationary. Do not pull up with your arms and shoulders but instead use your lower core to lift your legs. Concentrate on keeping your core tight during the entire movement. Bring your legs down in a controlled manner – just don't let them drop rapidly.

Reverse Cable Crunches (Upper Abs)

The reverse cable crunch is not usually performed with proper form. Do not use your arms to pull the weight down. Instead, concentrate on using your core to pull the weights down and you will develop a very strong upper abdominal area. You should also make sure that you perform the *full range* of motion and touch your elbows to your knees. If your arms get tired during a heavy lift then you are almost certainly depending too heavily on your arms instead of using your core abs to get the weights pulled down.

LOONIE CRUNCH

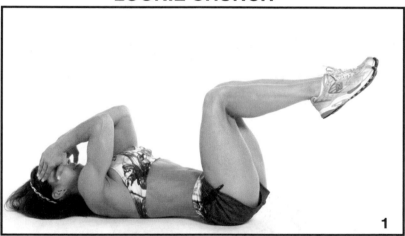

1. LOONIE CRUNCH START POSITION

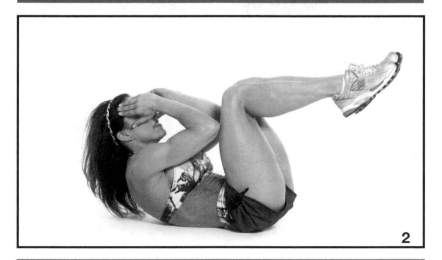

2. LOONIE CRUNCH FINISH POSITION

HANGING LEG RAISE

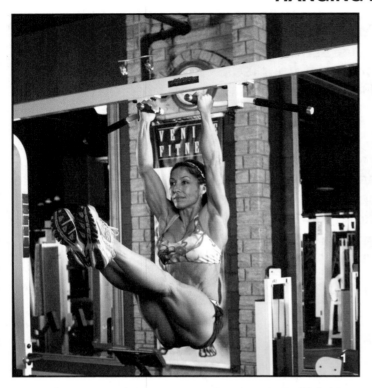

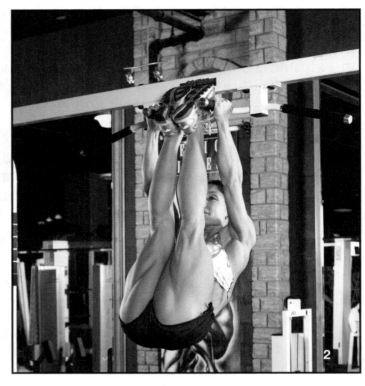

1. HANGING LEG RAISE TO HALFWAY

2. HANGING LEG RAISE FULL RANGE

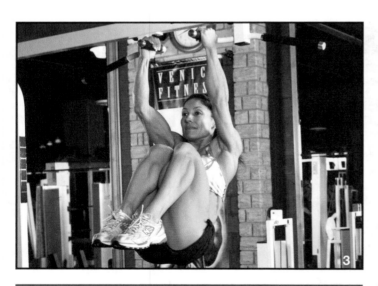

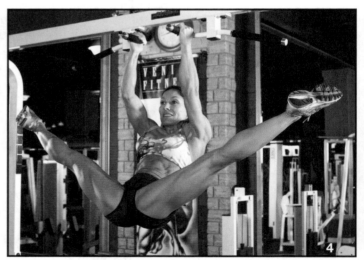

3. HANGING LEG RAISE KNEES TO CHEST - THEN KICK LEGS UP TO FULL RANGE TOP POSITION & RETURN DOWN SLOWLY

4. HANGING LEG RAISE - GO FULL RANGE TO THE TOP, AND THEN DO THE SPLITS AND RETURN DOWN SLOWLY

REVERSE CABLE CRUNCH

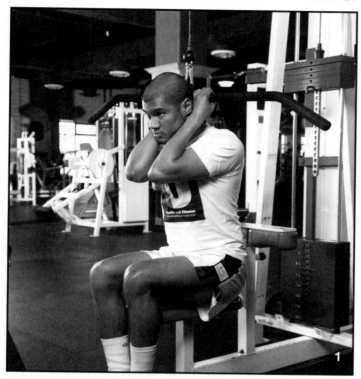

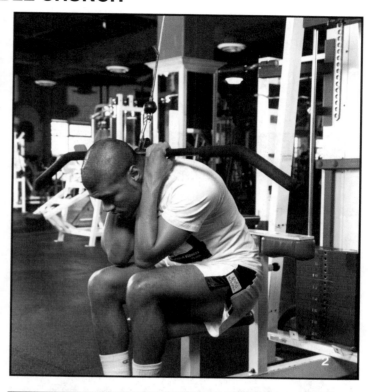

1. REVERSE CABLE CRUNCH WITH HEAVY WEIGHTS - START POSITION

2. REVERSE CABLE CRUNCH WITH HEAVY WEIGHTS - FINISH POSITION

Doug's Abdominal Routine

Just for your information, here is my daily ab routine at the age of 65 (please see photos to see how each exercise is performed):

- 10 repetitions of each of the four advanced hanging leg raises, or 20 to 25 repetitions of the full hanging leg raises up to the high bar

- 50 repetitions of advanced "loonie" crunches

- 3 sets of advanced reverse cable crunches with 20 reps of 100 pounds, 8 reps of 120 pounds, and 4 reps of 130 pounds

- 3 sets of flat bench crunches with 90 pounds, 135 pounds and 180 pounds holding for 30 to 60 seconds

If you think you already have great abs, just give this a whirl. When I asked eight time Canadian National Amateur Lightweight Boxing Champion Ibrahim Kamil to rate this specific routine on a difficulty scale from 1 to 10, he gave it a 15 !

Flat Bench Plate Crunch

This routine can be viewed on the ULTIMA website video. This is a highly difficult and risky routine that requires a rock-solid core and strong lower back.

Back Extensions

In order to ensure that you have a solid core from front to back, you need to exercise the lower back by doing back extensions, which are demonstrated below.

START POSITION

FINISH POSITION

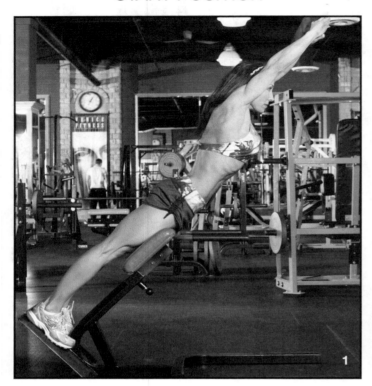

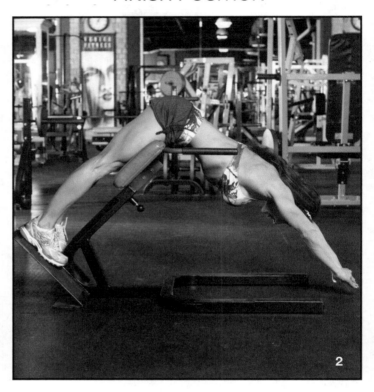

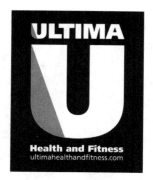

CHAPTER
15
CHEST EXERCISES

As mentioned in an earlier chapter, all weight training exercises should be done with smooth and controlled motions and only those body parts that are directly involved with lift should be in motion; the rest of your body should remain still.

For chest exercises you can alternate between a barbell and dumbells from week to week. As I mentioned earlier, machines provide a more stabile exercise environment but they will not properly work the stabilizer muscles if you are involved with competitive sports. Weigh the benefits and setbacks of machines carefully and choose which routine is best for your lifestyle.

You can choose three basic routines and three finishing routines each day using any one of the barbells, dumbbells or machines shown in the photos.

For barbell training, use a grip about shoulder width. The bar should come down to a point about halfway between your sternum and your chin, as shown in the photos.

BASIC ROUTINES

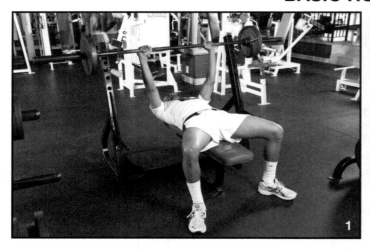

1. FLAT BENCH WITH BARBELL START POSITION

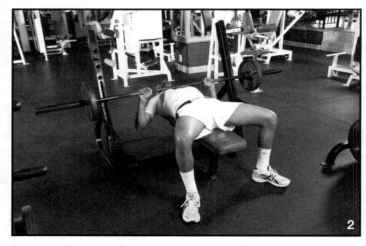

2. FLAT BENCH WITH BARBELL FINISH POSITION

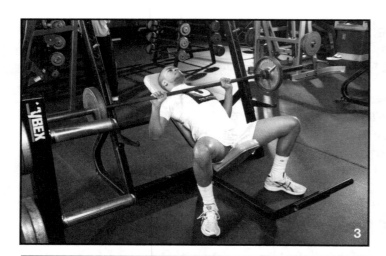

3. INCLINE BENCH FINISH POSITION – THE START POSITION IS THE SAME AS FOR FLAT BENCH

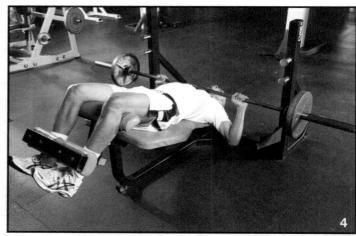

4. DECLINE BENCH FINISH POSITION – THE START POSITION IS THE SAME AS FOR FLAT BENCH

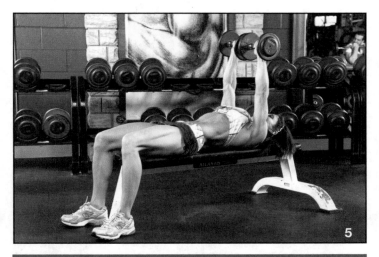

5. FLAT BENCH DUMBELL START POSITION

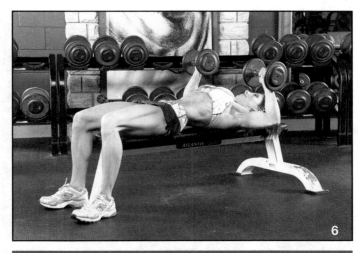

6. FLAT BENCH DUMBELL FINISH POSITION

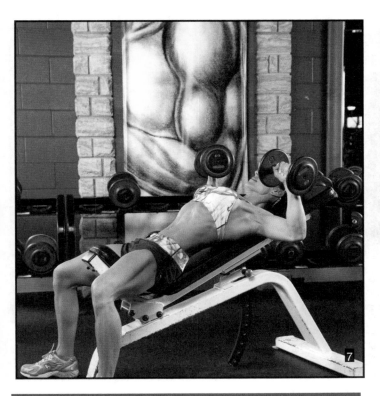

7. INCLINE BENCH DUMBELL FINISH POSITION – THE START POSITION IS THE SAME AS FOR FLAT BENCH

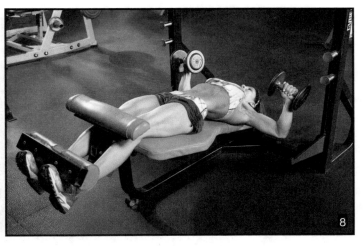

8. DECLINE BENCH DUMBELL FINISH POSITION – THE START POSITION IS THE SAME AS FOR FLAT BENCH

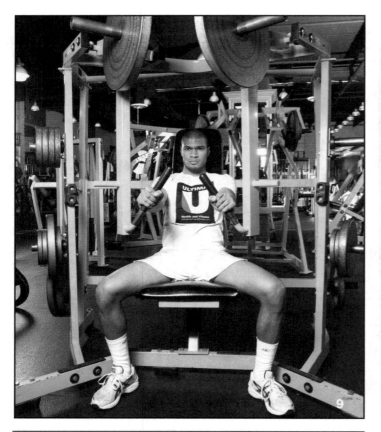

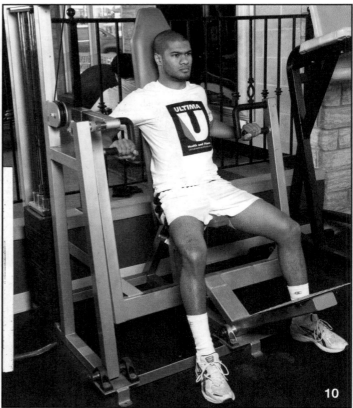

9. HAMMER MACHINE CHEST MACHINES HAVE THREE SEPARATE MODELS TO SIMULATE FLAT BENCH, INCLINE BENCH OR DECLINE BENCH AND CAN BE SUBSTITUTED FOR BARBELLS DUMBELLS

10. SEATED CHEST PRESS IS ANOTHER ALTERNATIVE TO DOING FLAT BENCH

FINISHING ROUTINES

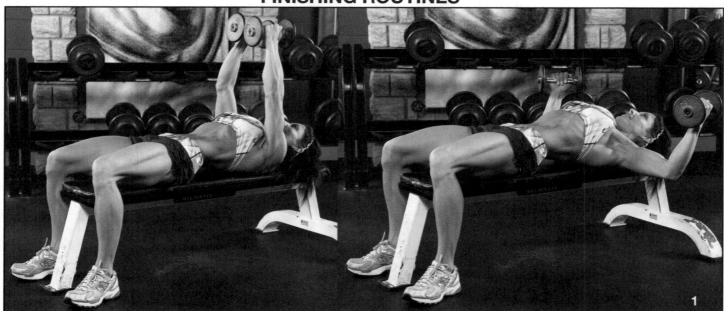

1. DUMBELL FLY START POSITION

1. DUMBELL FLY FINISH POSITION

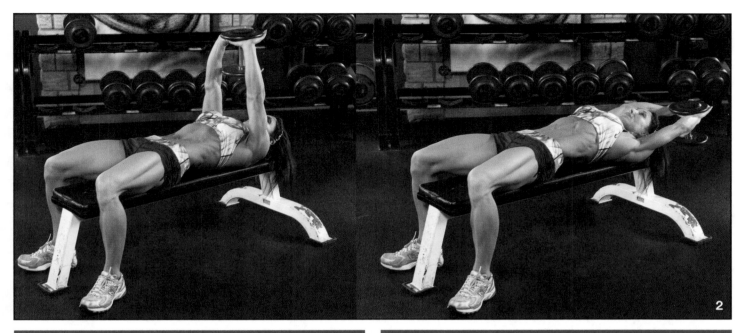

2. DUMBELL PULLOVER START POSITION

2. DUMBELL PULLOVER FINISH POSITION

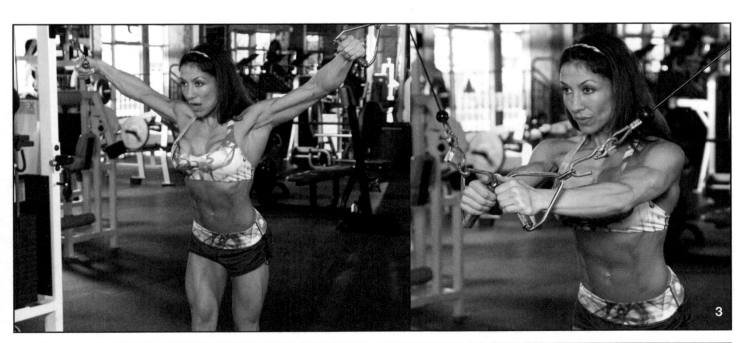

3. CABLE FLY START POSITION

2. CABLE FLY FINISH POSITION

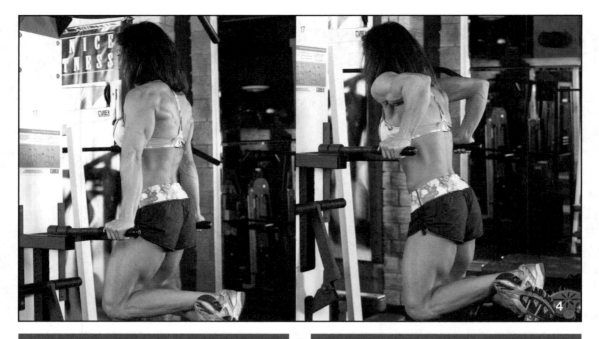

4. DIPS START POSITION

4. DIPS FINISH POSITION

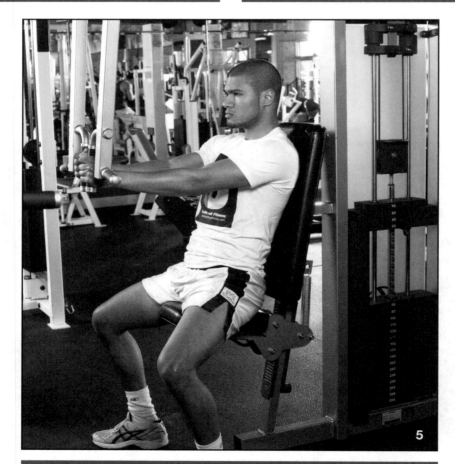

5. PECK DECK

SMITH MACHINE STOP POSITION PIN

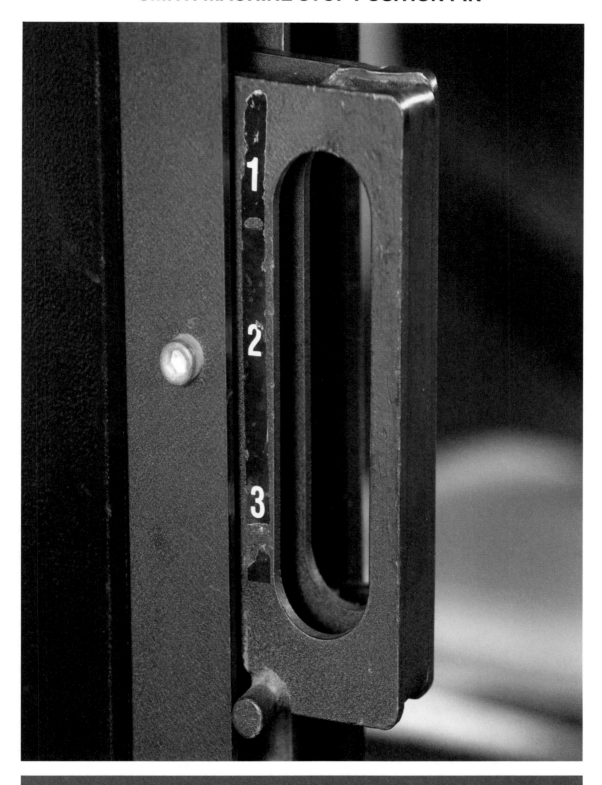

THE SMITH MACHINE MAY BE SUPPLIED WITH A STOP POSITION PIN WHICH PREVENTS WEIGHTS FROM GOING BELOW A FIXED POSITION THAT YOU CAN ESTABLISH BEFORE YOU START A LIFT. THIS IS A GREAT SAFETY FEATURE WHEN YOU ARE PERFORMING NEGATIVES OR LIFTING WEIGHTS WHICH YOU HAVE NEVER LIFTED BEFORE.

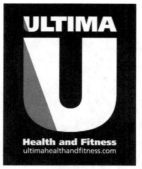

CHAPTER
16
BACK EXERCISES

Please perform the first three exercises in the photos in the order that they appear and then move on to the other exercises in an order of your choosing. When you are performing all back exercises, you need to ensure that you are performing a *full extension*, or *full range of motion* to be most effective. While training using a half range is much easier, it does not help you to progress and develop your muscles properly; you need to use a full extension. Initially, you may have to use a machine that assists you in the lift, but in a few weeks or months you should be able to complete the routines shown below with no assistance.

On the lat pull down cable routine, concentrate on keeping your back straight and do not lean far back to pull down heavier weights. You might think you are getting stronger, but you are not using the proper muscle group when you perform this exercise by leaning backward.

The first three back exercises (chins and dead lift) are the most important to perform and the others can be used as finishing routines.

START POSITION	FINISH POSITION

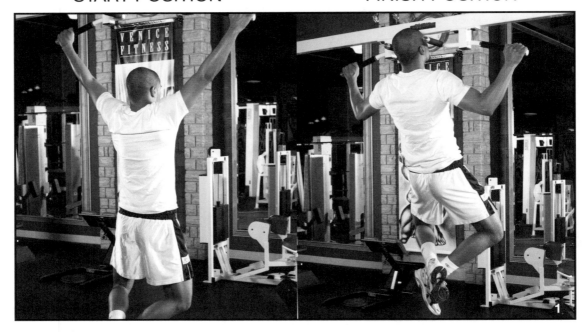

1. WIDE GRIP CHINS - PRONATED GRIP WITH PALMS FACING AWAY FROM YOU

START POSITION	FINISH POSITION

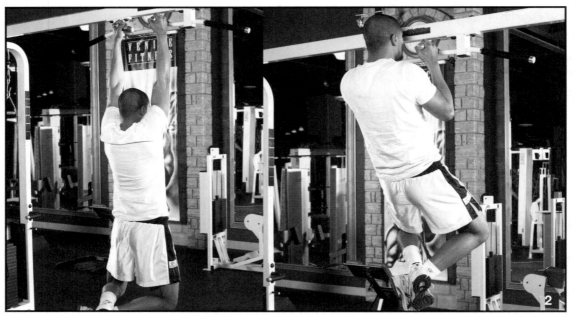

2. NARROW GRIP CHINS - PALMS OF HANDS FACING INWARD

START POSITION   FINISH POSITION

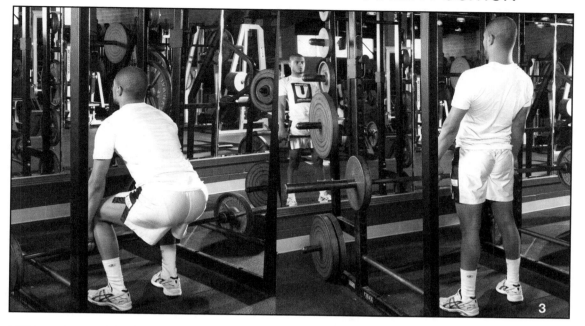

3. DEAD LIFT START POSITION – NOTE THE POSITION OF LEGS AND BACK IN THIS PHOTO; DEAD LIFT FINISH POSITION – NOTE ARCHED BACK AND CHEST OUT

START POSITION   FINISH POSITION

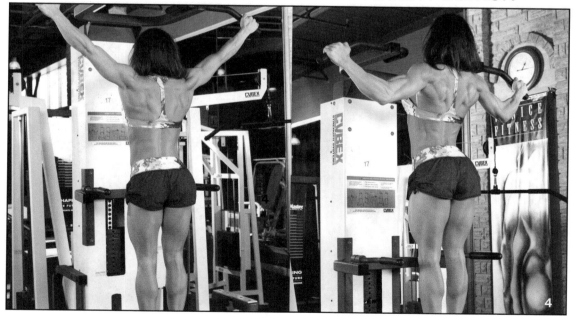

4. WIDE GRIP CHINS PRONATED GRIP WITH ASSISTANCE FROM THE MACHINE; IN THESE PHOTOS, A MACHINE IS BEING USED TO REDUCE THE EFFORT TO PERFORM THE EXERCISE. YOU CAN DECIDE HOW EASY OR HOW HARD TO MAKE THE ROUTINE BY SIMPLY ADJUSTING A PIN.

START POSITION

FINISH POSITION

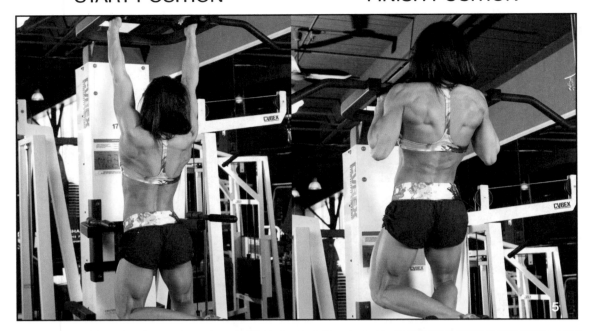

5. NARROW GRIP CHINS WITH PALMS FACING INWARD AND ASSISTANCE FROM THE MACHINE; IN THESE PHOTOS, A MACHINE IS BEING USED TO REDUCE THE EFFORT TO PERFORM THE EXERCISE. YOU CAN DECIDE HOW EASY OR HOW HARD TO MAKE THE ROUTINE BY SIMPLY ADJUSTING A PIN.

START POSITION

FINISH POSITION

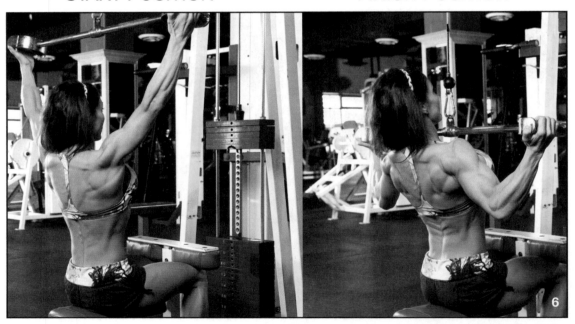

6. CABLE PULL DOWN. YOU CAN SUBSTITUTE ANOTHER SHORT BAR TO SIMULATE A CLOSE GRIP ROUTINE.

START POSITION   FINISH POSITION

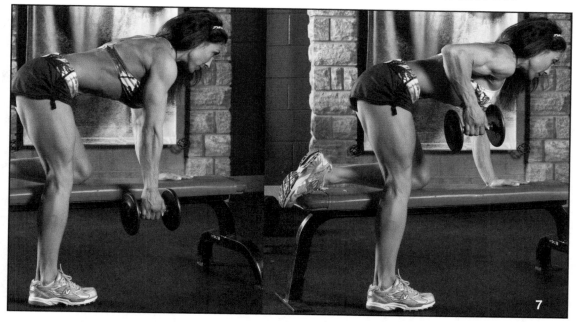

7. SINGLE ARM DUMBELL LIFT.

START POSITION   FINISH POSITION

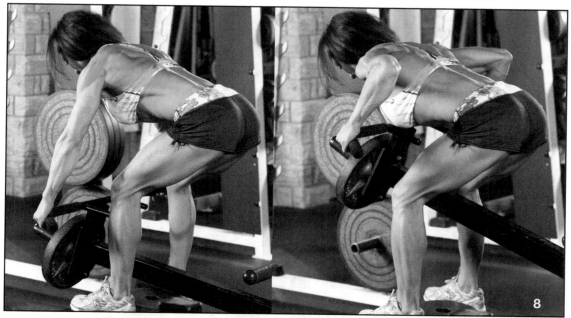

8. T-BAR LIFT.

START POSITION FINISH POSITION

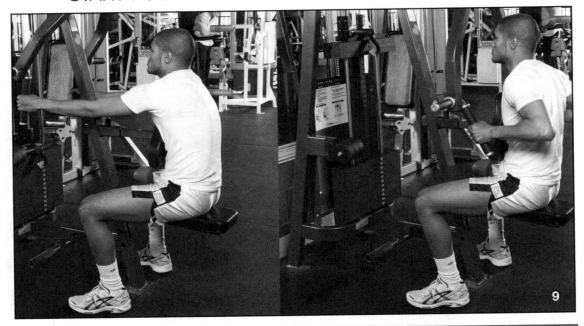

9. SEATED CABLE ROW. THERE ARE ALSO MANY OTHER TYPES OF SEATED ROWING MACHINES IN MOST GYMS USING EITHER CABLES OR WEIGHTS. TRY THEM ALL AND SEE WHICH ONE WORKS BEST FOR YOU.

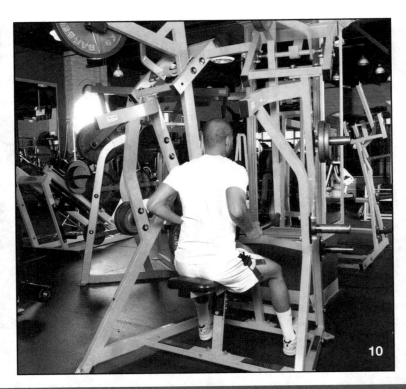

10. THERE ARE SEVERAL TYPES OF HAMMER MACHINES AVAILABLE IN MANY GYMS WHICH CAN PERFORM A VARIETY OF BACK ROUTINES FOR DIFFERENT BACK MUSCLES.

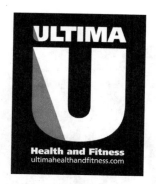

CHAPTER
17
SHOULDER EXERCISES

Please ensure that you perform shoulder warm up routines each day. These warm up routines can be done with no rest between sets because so you are not using heavy weights. As with back exercises, you need to use a full range of motion on all exercise routines to be most effective.

I do not recommend doing shoulder presses behind the neck, as I have witnessed a number of experienced trainers get injured by performing this routine. I recommend that you stick with a front of the chest military press instead.

There are a variety of Hammer Machines that can be substituted for the exercises shown below.

START POSITION FINISH POSITION

START POSITION   FINISH POSITION

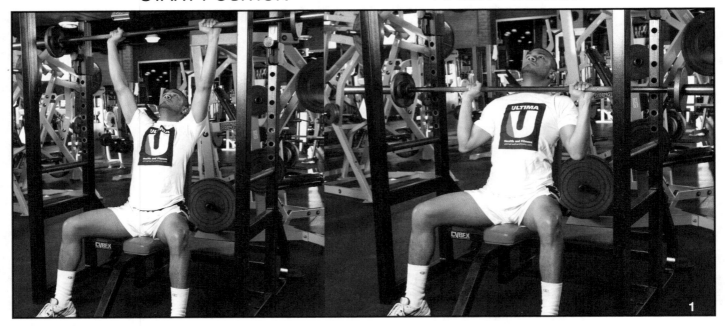

1. SEATED BARBELL FRONT SHOULDER PRESS. YOU CAN SUBSTITUTE DUMBELLS FOR THIS EXERCISE AND EITHER BE SEATED OR STANDING WHEN YOU ARE USING THE DUMBELLS.

START POSITION   FINISH POSITION

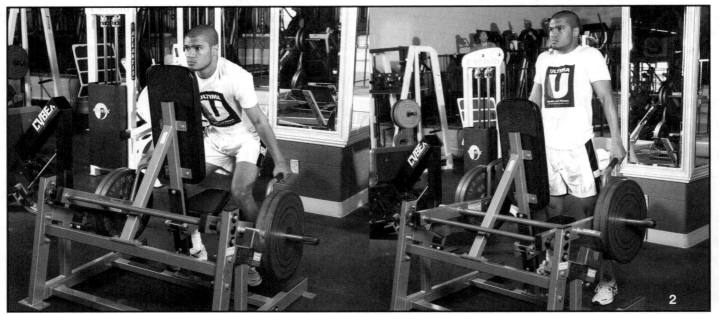

2. SHOULDER SHRUG. YOU CAN ALSO USE DUMBELLS OR BARBELLS TO DO THIS EXERCISE.

START POSITION   FINISH POSITION

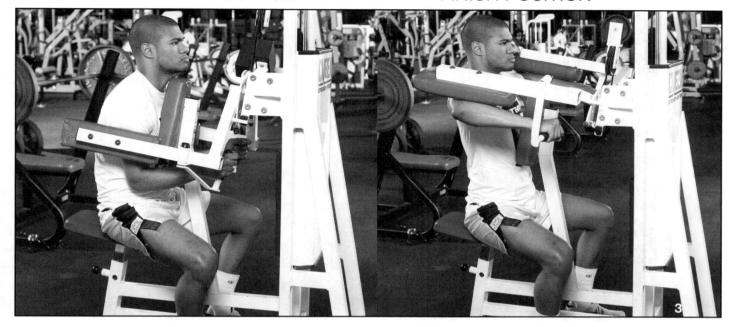

3. LATERAL SHOULDER RAISE.

START POSITION   FINISH POSITION

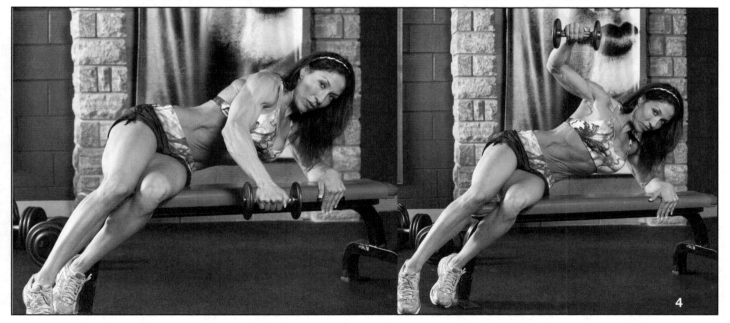

4. LYING REAR DELT.

START POSITION   FINISH POSITION

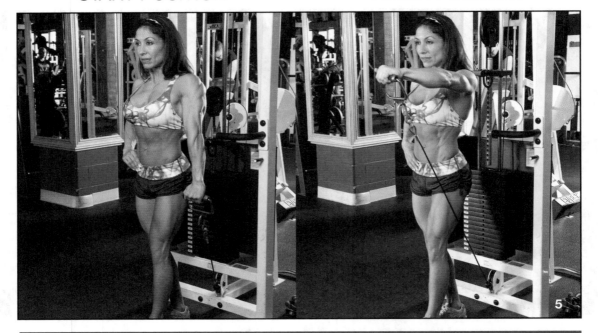

5. FRONT SHOULDER CABLE RAISE.

START POSITION   FINISH POSITION

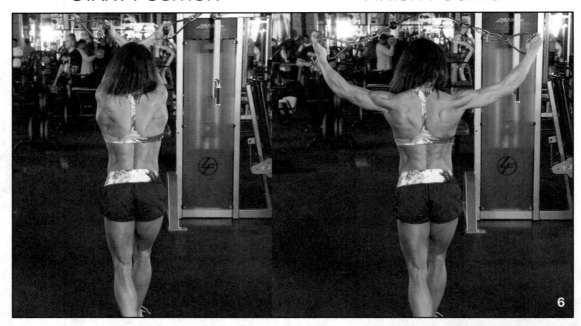

6. HIGH CABLE CROSSOVERS. NOTE THE POSITION OF THE ARMS AT THE END OF THE ROUTINE, ABOVE THE HEAD.

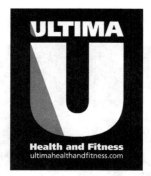

CHAPTER
18
Bicep and Triceps Exercises

As mentioned previously in the book, you are able to perform a bicep routine followed immediately by a triceps routine before you take a rest. In performing these exercises back-to-back, you can increase productivity and reduce your training time for these body parts. When performing these exercises, *do not move any other part of your body* in order to be most effective. I find that bending my knees slightly on any standing routine helps to keep my body stable and motionless during the exercise. When performing triceps routines, keep the elbows in tight/close to your body and *keep your elbows still*. Please ensure that you are doing a full range of motion when performing your routines, as shown in the accompanying photos.

Choose four of each bicep and triceps routines, performing the more difficult routines first, followed by routines that call for single arm work.

START POSITION	FINISH POSITION

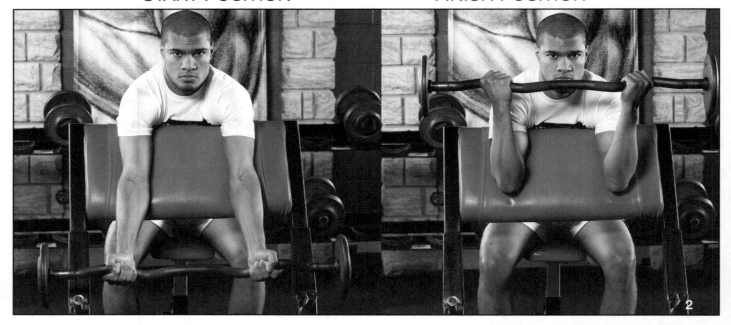

1. DOUBLE ARM HIGH CABLE CURL. NOTE THE POSITION OF THE HANDS TO THE SIDES OF THE TEMPLE AT THE FINISH POSITION.

START POSITION	FINISH POSITION

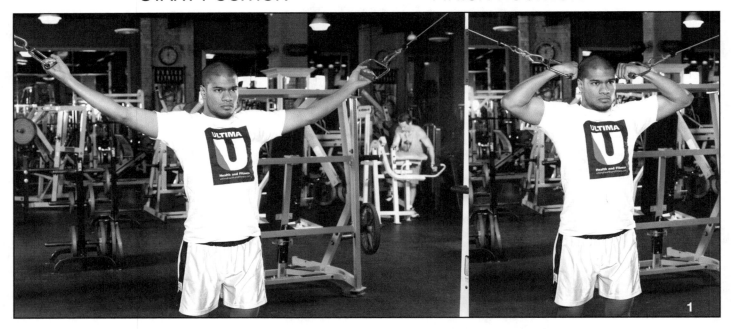

2. PREACHER CURL.

START POSITION   FINISH POSITION

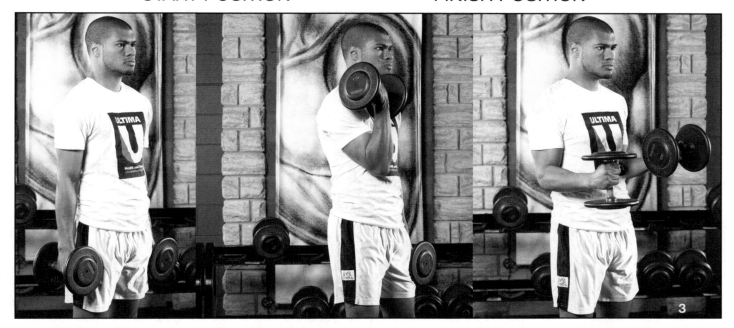

3. COMBINATION TWISTING CURL UP AND HAMMER POSITION DOWN - STAGE ONE, BRING ONE ARM UP IN A TWISTING MOTION AND THEN, TURN THE WEIGHTS TO A HAMMER POSITION. AS YOU BRING THE WEIGHTS DOWN, BEGIN THE MOVEMENT UP WITH THE OPPOSITE ARM SO THAT THEY MEET HALF-WAY. REPEAT THE MOVEMENT WITH THE SECOND ARM. KEEP THE REST OF YOUR BODY STILL AT ALL TIMES.

START POSITION   FINISH POSITION

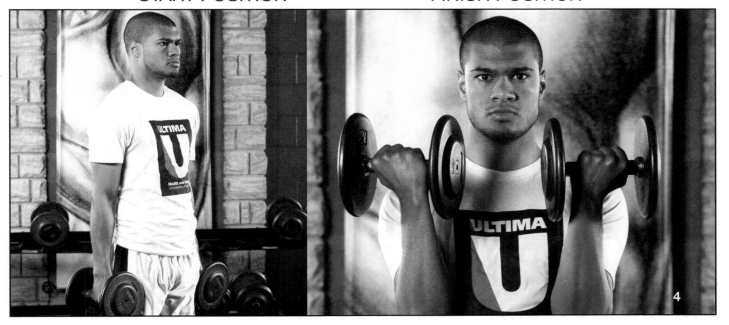

4. STANDARD DUMBELL CURLS.

START POSITION	FINISH POSITION

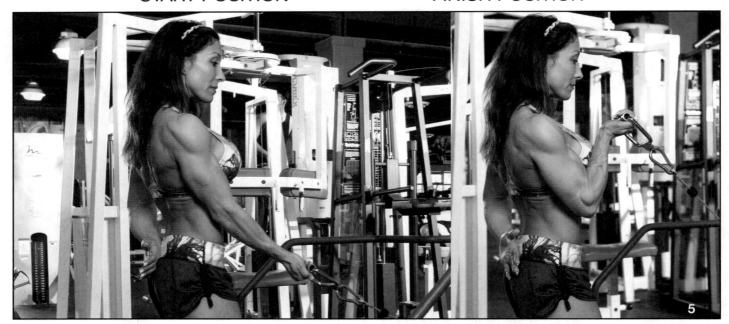

5. SINGLE ARM CABLE CURL. NOTE, YOU STAND A FEW FEET AWAY FROM THE MACHINE SO THAT THE WEIGHTS HAVE ALREADY BEEN LIFTED AS YOU BEGIN THE EXERCISE. THIS PUTS CONSTANT STRESS ON THE BICEP DURNG THE ENTIRE ROUTINE.

START POSITION	FINISH POSITION

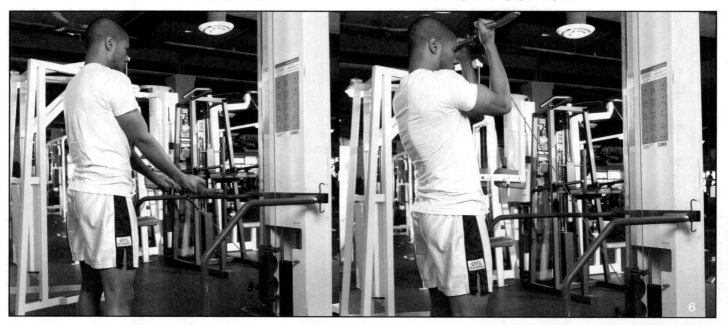

6. DOUBLE ARM HIGH CABLE TO FOREHEAD. NOTE, YOU STAND A FEW FEET AWAY FROM THE MACHINE SO THAT THE WEIGHTS HAVE ALREADY BEEN LIFTED AS YOU BEGIN THE EXERCISE. THIS PUTS CONSTANT STRESS ON THE BICEP DURING THE ENTIRE ROUTINE. CONCENTRATE ON KEEPING THE BODY STILL AND THE BODY AT ARM'S LENGTH AWAY DURING THE ENTIRE ROUTINE. NOTE THE FINISH POSITION WITH THE BAR AT YOUR FOREHEAD. YOU CAN SUBSTITUTE A ROPE FOR THIS ROUTINE.

START POSITION   FINISH POSITION

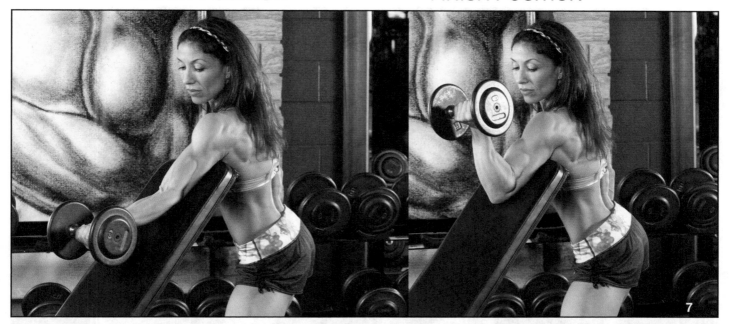

7. SINGLE ARM STANDING INCLINE BENCH CURL. NOTE THAT THE THUMB SHOULD BE PLACED UNDER THE BAR, ALONG WITH YOUR FINGERS, KEEP YOUR ARMPIT LOCKED IN PLACE AT THE TOP OF THE BENCH AND BRING THE WEIGHT DOWN TO ABOUT HALF AN INCH ABOVE THE BENCH - IT SHOULD NOT TOUCH THE PAD, THEREBY KEEPING CONSTANT STRESS ON THE BICEP.

START POSITION   FINISH POSITION

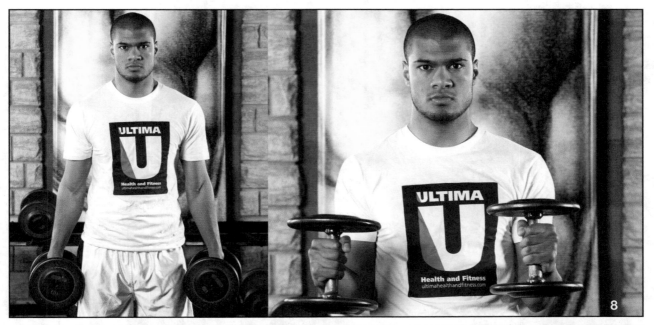

8. HAMMER CURLS HELP TO DEVELOP YOUR FOREARMS.

START POSITION

FINISH POSITION

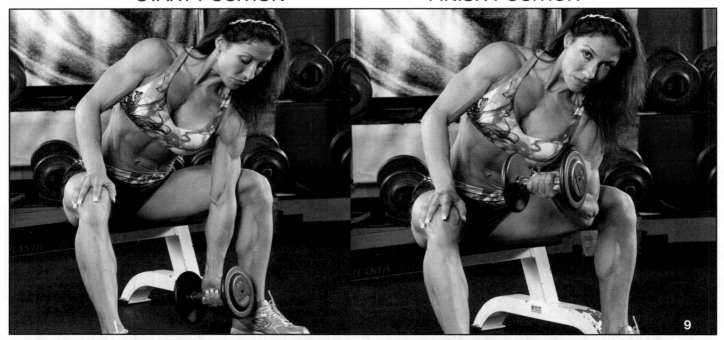

9. SINGLE ARM CONCENTRATION CURL.

START POSITION

FINISH POSITION

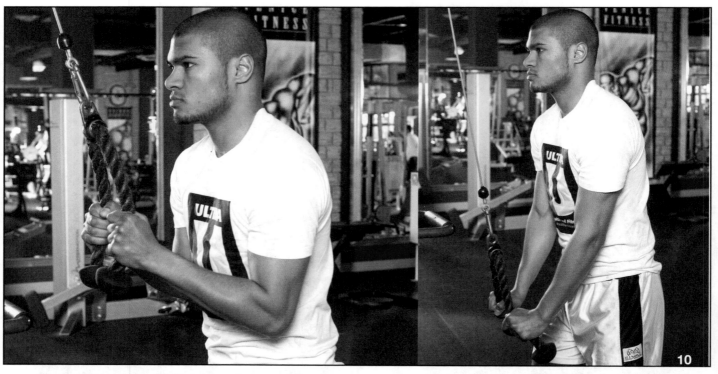

10. ROPE TRICEPS START POSITION; ROPE TRICEPS FINISH POSITION. NOTE THE POSITIONING OF THE HANDS IN THE MIDDLE PART OF THE ROPE – THIS REQUIRES MORE HAND STRENGTH AND THE HANDS SHOULD REMAIN IN THIS POSITION THROUGHOUT THE MOVEMENT. AT THE END OF EACH MOVEMENT, JUST BEFORE THE FINISH, TWIST YOUR WRISTS TO THE OUTSIDE. YOU CAN SUBSTITUTE EITHER A SHORT STRAIGHT BAR OR A V-BAR FOR THE ROPE.

START POSITION   FINISH POSITION

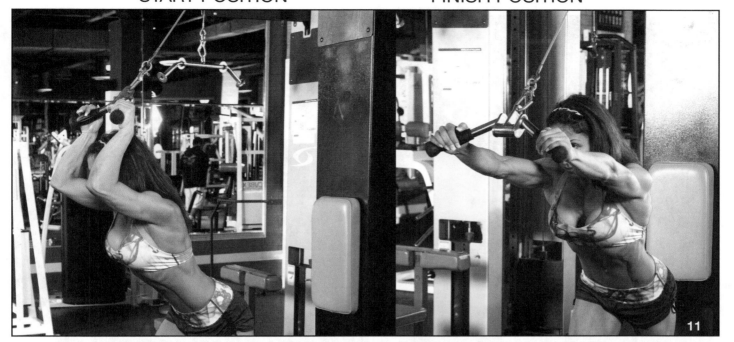

11. OVERHEAD CABLE TRICEP START POSITION; OVERHEAD CABLE TRICEP FINISH POSITION
KEEP ELBOWS IN TIGHT AND USE FULL RANGE OF MOTION. NOTE POSITION OF FEET AWAY FROM MACHINE TO
ENSURE CONSTANT STRESS ON THE MUSCLE GROUP. YOU CAN USE EITHER THE ROPE, V-BAR OR SHORT BAR.

START POSITION   FINISH POSITION

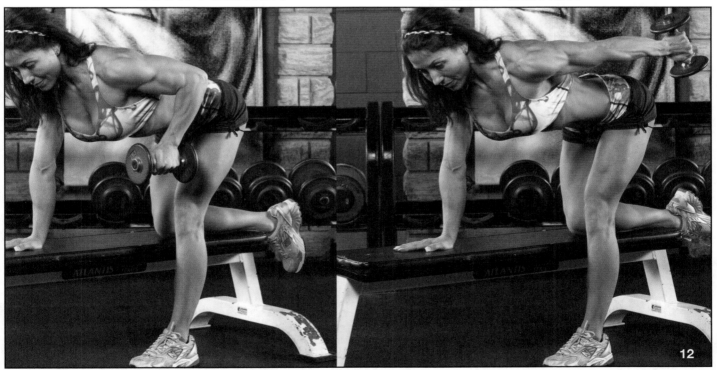

12. DUMBELL KICKBACK.

START POSITION   FINISH POSITION

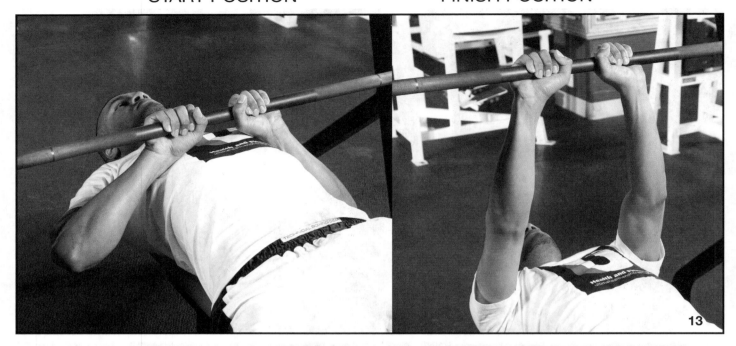

13. CLOSE GRIP BARBELL TRICEPS.

START POSITION   FINISH POSITION

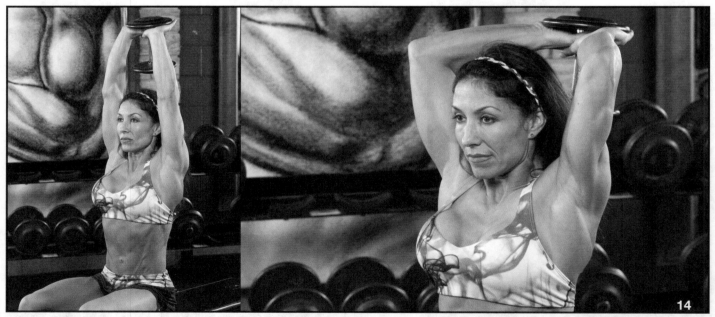

14. SEATED TRICEP DUMBELL.

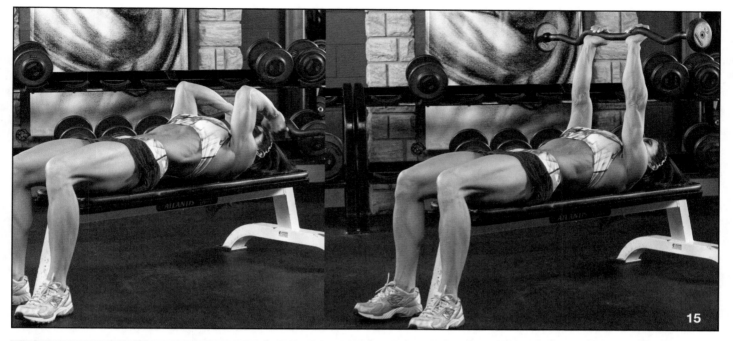

15. SKULL CRUSHER.

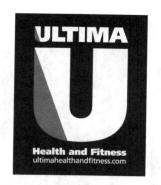

CHAPTER
19
LEG EXERCISES

I have always done my leg exercises in the following sequence:

1. Abductors
2. Calf raises
3. Hamstring exercises
4. Leg extensions
5. Squats and/or leg press
6. Lunges

Another option is to do the squats and/or leg press first. Once again, you need to experiment to see what works best for yourself. You should perform all the exercises shown on each training day.

Make absolutely certain that you use the form shown in the pictures for squats and do not go beyond 90 degrees. Touching the ground with your behind puts tremendous and unnecessary stress on your knees and can cause serious knee injuries. One gym member who used to squat over 500 pounds this way destroyed both his knees and required major surgery to repair torn cartilage. Don't be another victim of injury due to improper form when weightlifting.

Start your leg training with light weights and gradually add weights each week to build your muscle strength.

START POSITION   FINISH POSITION

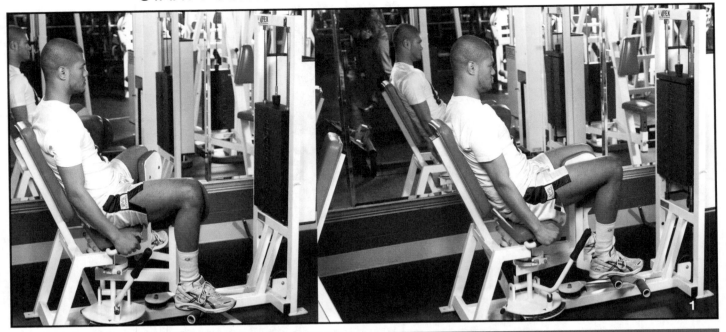

1. ABDUCTOR STRETCH. YOU NEED TO SQUEEZE THE PADS TOGETHER SO THAT THEY TOUCH. SET THE MACHINE AT THE START POSITION TO AS WIDE AS POSSIBLE AS IS COMFORTABLE IN ORDER TO GET THE MOST STRETCH. THERE IS ALSO A SIMILAR DESIGNED MACHINE THAT YOU CAN PERFORM THIS EXERCISE BY PUSHING PADS TO THE OUTSIDE, WITH YOUR LEGS.

START POSITION   FINISH POSITION

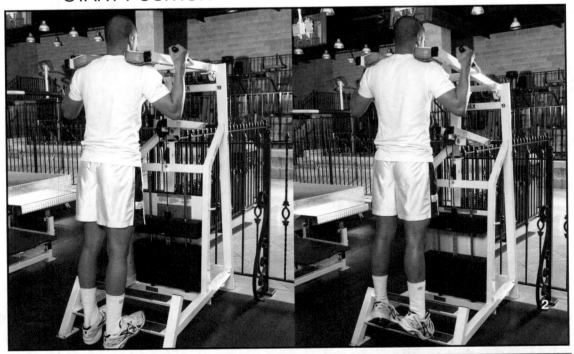

2. CALF RAISE. THERE ARE MANY DIFFERENT TYPES OF CALF MACHINES THAT CAN BE USED, SUCH AS A SEATED CALF MACHINE.

START POSITION	FINISH POSITION

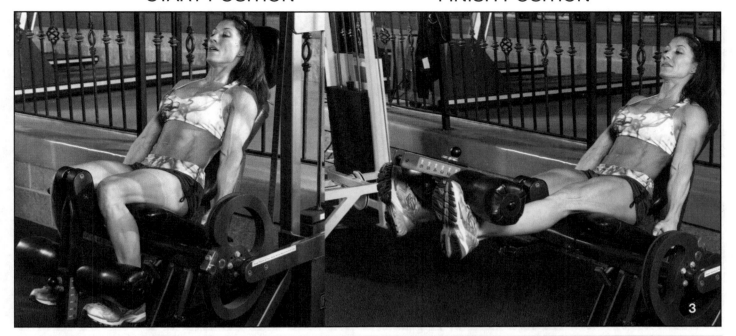

3. LEG EXTENSIONS. THIS EXERCISE TRAINS THE QUADRACEP MUSCLES ABOVE THE KNEE TO THE THIGH.

START POSITION	FINISH POSITION

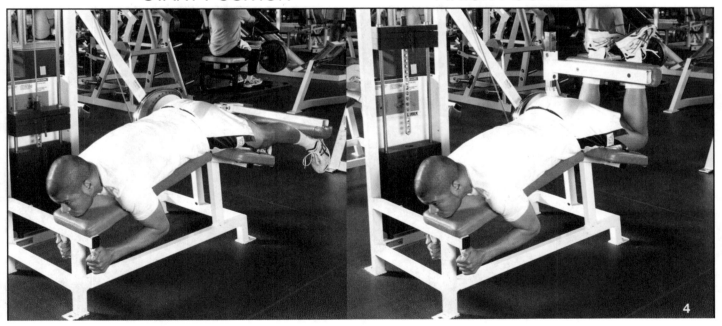

4. HAMSTRING CURL. THIS EXERCISE TRAINS THE HAMSTRING MUSCLE ON THE BACK OF YOUR LEG. YOU SHOULD TRY TO CURL THE BAR AS MUCH AS POSSIBLE SO THAT THE HEELS OF YOUR FEET COME AS CLOSE TO YOUR BEHIND AS POSSIBLE. THERE ARE ALSO SINGLE LEG STANDING CURL MACHINES AVAIBLE AT MANY GYMS.

START POSITION　　　　　FINISH POSITION

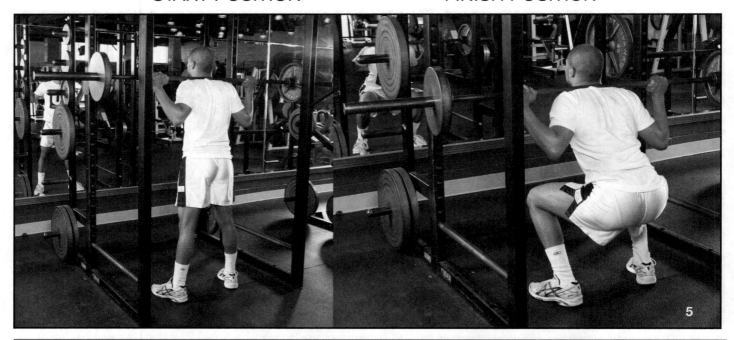

5. SQUAT POSITION. NOTE HEAD UP, LOOKING FORWARD, ARCHED BACK AND 90 DEGREE ANGLE LEGS IN THE FINISH POSITION.

START POSITION　　　　　FINISH POSITION

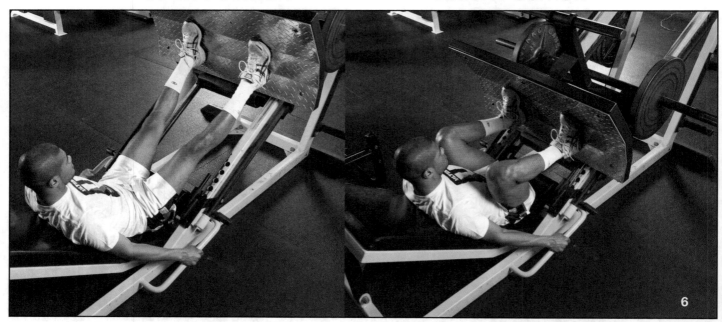

6. LEG PRESS START POSITION; LEG PRESS FINISH POSITION. POSITIONING OF EQUIPMENT AND LEGS IS CRITICAL TO GET THE MOST OUT OF THIS ROUTINE. SET SEAT BACK AS FAR BACK AS POSSIBLE AND SET THE STOP PINS ON THE SIDE RAILS TO THE LOWEST POSITION TO ENSURE MAXIMUM RANGE OF MOTION. KEEP LEGS SHOULDER WIDTH APART AND BRING THE WEIGHT DOWN TO ABOUT HALF AN INCH ABOVE THE STOP POSITION. DO NOT BOUNCE THE WEIGHTS OFF THE STOP POSITION. NOTE THE POSITION OF THE FEET – SETTING THEM LOWER MAKES FOR A MORE DIFFICULT ROUTINE.

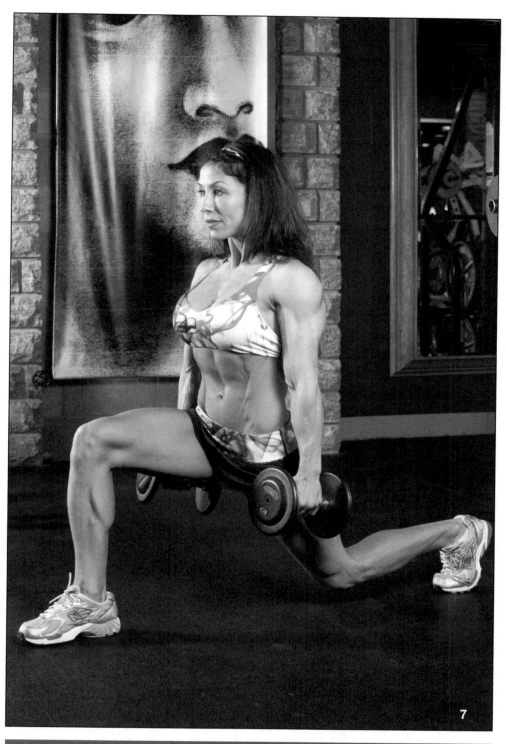

7. LUNGES CAN BE DONE MOVING EITHER FORWARD OR BACKWARDS – MANY TRAINERS USE THIS EXERCISE AS A "MUST DO" BY THEIR CLIENTS.

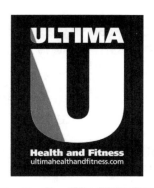

CHAPTER
20
CARDIOVASCULAR EXERCISES

There are a multitude of choices for cardio exercises ranging from walking, running, skipping, bicycling, swimming, boxing, tennis, treadmills, Stairmasters and so forth. I have tried all of them, and for me the Stairmaster 4400-4600 and boxing were my top choices for maximum stamina. My training partner for years was a former professional football player and he used the treadmill and elliptical machines on a regular basis. After he used the Stairmaster machine at a difficult level, he commented that the treadmill and elliptical machines were "a walk in the park" in comparison. Boxing clubs often offer group classes that involve good training, but no physical sparring. While these are my personal recommendations for cardio exercises, I recommend that you try out a number of options to see what works best for you and do what you enjoy performing the most.

Before you get started, you need to see your physician to ensure that you are physically capable of performing strenuous cardio work without causing injury. I would also recommend an annual physical exam including blood work each year for the future to ensure good health is maintained. Physician visits can also be helpful in monitoring improvements made to your health and fitness. You will be astounded at the improvements that can be made to your body in a year if you follow the course of action recommended in this book for both nutrition and exercise.

In developing a cardio routine on any one of the cardio machines available in most local gyms, there are four stages you can follow to ensure your success. You need to slowly but surely build up your stamina and challenge yourself to do better each week. It may require several months to move from one stage to the next.

- Stage 1: Start off at a low level of intensity and use three 10 minute sessions, with a 1 minute break between each session. Slowly increase the intensity for each of these 10 minute sessions, but keep the break time the same.

- Stage 2: Change the routine to two 15 minute sessions and increase the intensity of the sessions over time. Still use a 1 minute break in between sessions.

- Stage 3: The next step is a 20 minute session followed by a 10 minute session. As before, increase the intensity over time and give yourself a 1 minute rest between the first and second session.

- Stage 4: Finally, go to a 30 minute session with no rest, and keep increasing the intensity.

No matter what type of cardio exercise you end up choosing, please continue to challenge yourself. As the saying goes, the sky is the limit.

It took me a year of consistent hard work to finally endure a difficult 30-minute routine, but the rewards were worth the effort. A twenty-eight year old semi-professional soccer player tried my most difficult 30-minute routine that I was able to complete at fifty-seven years old. He lasted under 7 minutes. That is how good you can get when you take the time and effort to build your endurance.

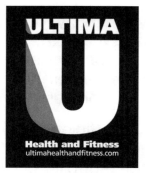

CHAPTER
21
CLOSING SUMMARY

In closing, I'd like to recap all of the major fundamentals from this book that will help you to make a permanent and lasting change to your health, fitness and well being.

1. You need to remember the five keys to fitness, which are: patience, consistency in your nutrition and exercise habits, hard work, a proper nutrition program, and a proper exercise/training program. I sincerely hope that this book has given you the necessary tools to achieve all of those goals.

2. You can not buy your health. The benefits of regular exercise have been documented and supported by leading health experts around the world, regardless of the age you begin. You need to establish an exercise program that will provide you with the tools to achieve proper body weight, flexibility, strength and endurance. Any exercise program you use should provide exercise for all body parts and include cardiovascular training.

3. There is a worldwide obesity and diabetes epidemic that can be solved primarily through proper nutrition and exercise.

4. Water is the single most important ingredient you ingest. Make sure that you are drinking clean water, which can be obtained through the use of water distillers or reverse osmosis equipment. Save yourself money and reduce your environmental impact by eliminating plastic water bottles and utilizing stainless steel bottles in their place.

5. I have provided you with healthy and tasty food plans that can assist you in reaching your targeted weight goals. Please make the effort to post the list of basic nutrition and exercise principles on your refrigerator as a daily reminder of what you need to do to change your life for the better. Remember, carbohydrates are for fuel or energy, and protein is for building muscle or power.

6. The food you eat may not supply sufficient nutrients for your body. If you decide to utilize vitamin and mineral supplements to top up your daily needs, I suggest you use combination packs from reputable suppliers. These suppliers should have a proven track record regarding the quality of their products, a demonstrated knowledge of how much of each supplement is required for your body, and how supplements interact with one another.

7. You need to remember to train without pain, and to ensure that you get adequate sleep on a quality bed.

8. History has provided us with countless world champions who succeeded without the crutch of performance enhancing drugs or other techniques like blood doping. Avoid the pitfalls and dangers that these substances and techniques will bring, and remember that you should never underestimate your own abilities to achieve your personal goals.

9. I have provided you with an array of training routines for each of your individual body parts and by utilizing these routines, you can improve your body and your health. There are machines that can be used in place of free weights, which may provide you with a safer workout environment. Choose a program that works for you but ensure that the program meets all of your needs and goals.

Try your best, make no excuses and you will gain self respect and the respect of others. Never fear failure, but prove to yourself and others that you can and will overcome the health and fitness challenges that life brings. Do not hesitate to get professional help if you have an eating disorder, if you need help in training, or if you need advice regarding nutrition. With the guidance of this book, you can - and will - reach your fitness and nutrition goals so long as you maintain discipline, consistency and perseverance. Make health and fitness a top priority - your life depends on it.

Best wishes for a long and healthy life to you and your family.

Doug Fulford

May 2011

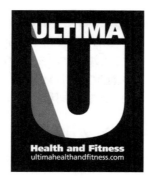

Dedications

This book is dedicated to the many people who inspired me to step up and perform well beyond my perceived limits, and to achieve much more than I ever imagined in my life.

To my Mom and Dad, who provided a home filled with love, peace, laughter, harmony, caring, guidance, and happiness. They taught me the principles of honesty, loyalty, and hard work, and to be a good and fair person. It was this foundation that provided me the basis for my conduct for the rest of my life.

To my brother Bob and his wife April, without whom this book would never have been produced. They provided much needed support when I needed it most and made tremendous personal sacrifices, especially of their own time, to help our family. I owe them for life.

To my ancestors, whose collective history is very special to me. I believe each member of my grandparents' four families has touched me with a little piece of their distinct personalities, and I feel blessed by all their influences. They are a magic part of my heritage and have been of great significance in the journey of my life.

To my paternal grandfather Edward Fulford, who survived through years of trench warfare in WW1. Anyone who has ever read stories of condition in the trenches of WW1 knows full well what it took to survive those horrendous circumstances.

To my maternal grandfather, Alexander Albert MacLeod, a brilliant, disciplined intellectual who fought for human rights. He was associated with the Communist movement in

Canada in the 1930s and later sat as a member of the Labour Party in the Ontario Legislature from 1943 to 1951. He held such respect that he was appointed as a consultant to the Ontario Human Rights Commission in 1960. He also was also involved with naming the busiest highway in Canada, to the "Macdonald-Cartier Freeway," after two of the forefathers of Canada. The term "401" was not acceptable to him!

To my paternal grandmother Lucy Pretty, who became a single divorced mother in the 1930s- one can only imagine how difficult it must have been to have dealt with that stigma in those days when it was not accepted. To her father, "Dapper" Daniel Pretty whose determination led him to walk over 250 miles from Hopetown to Toronto at age 16 to begin his career as a shoemaker. To his great-grandfather Daniel Pretty, who marched with the 76th Regiment of Foot of England and came to Canada to fight in the war against America in the fall of 1814, eventually settling in Canada after the Treaty of Ghent.

Special consideration is given to my great-grandfather Rufus Lawson Hicks (nicknamed "Rufus the Red"). Rufus demonstrated unwavering mental and physical courage over his entire lifetime. He persevered in the face of the losses of three of his four children, and one grandchild (my mother) to tragic accidents, as well as the loss of his wife to cancer in her latter years. His youngest son Ernest (nicknamed Wiggy) was hit by a truck and killed. His only daughter (my grandmother), burned to death when a woodstove exploded. Rufus carried the scars of burns to his arms to his grave, in trying to put out the flames. Then, his grand-daughter (my mother), whom he adored, was killed by a drunk driver. Near the end of his life, another son, Byron, died after he fell into a highway snow blower and had his arm and leg amputated. No one deserves to suffer so much personal grief over a lifetime. He was the toughest man I ever met, both physically and mentally, and yet he remained a humble, kind, and gentle man to the end. He is my personal hero, and I have a picture of him working in his fields, with the caption of my own words to reflect his life: "Hard work and perseverance never hurt anyone". I have always tried to carry on my life with this philosophy.

To the thousands of black jazz and R&B musicians and singers who lifted my spirits and brought peace to my soul in many troubled times. Your music inspired me beyond words and when I was way down, you brought me back up.

To my former fellow employees and business partner Burke Seitz, who for over 25 years supported me in every manner possible. It was the best overall business team that I have ever had the privilege to work with, and I could never have accomplished what was done without your help.

To my good friends, who have always been there in good times and bad.

Finally, to my wife Annemarie and my daughters Julie and Stephanie, as well as my grandson Cooper, whom I all love so much. Despite all the struggles, we have had so many wonderful memories that will never be forgotten.